STRONGER ABS AND BACK

Dean Brittenham, MS
Athletic Director
Shiley Athletic Elite Program

Greg Brittenham, MS
Strength and Conditioning Coach
New York Knicks

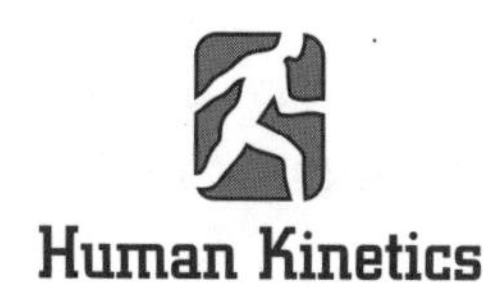

Human Kinetics

Library of Congress Cataloging-in-Publication Data

Brittenham, Dean, 1931-
Stronger abs and back / Dean Brittenham, Greg Brittenham.
p. cm.
ISBN: 0-88011-558-0
1. Exercise. 2. Abdomen--Muscles. 3. Back. I. Brittenham, Greg. II. Title.
GV508.B75 1997 96-48346
613.7'1--DC21 CIP

ISBN: 0-88011-558-0

Developmental Editor: Elaine Mustain; **Assistant Editor:** Susan Moore-Kruse; **Editorial Assistant:** Amy Carnes; **Copyeditor:** Bonnie Pettifor; **Proofreader:** Pam Johnson; **Graphic Designer:** Judy Henderson; **Graphic Artist:** Yvonne Winsor; **Photo Editor:** Boyd LaFoon; **Cover Designer:** Jack Davis; **Photographers (cover):** Ray Malace and D. Graham/H. Armstrong Roberts; **Photographer (interior):** John Sann; **Illustrator:** Patrick Griffin; **Mac Artist:** Sara Wolfsmith; **Printer:** United Graphics

Human Kinetics books are available at special discounts for bulk purchase. Special editions or book excerpts can also be created to specification. For details, contact the Special Sales Manager at Human Kinetics.

Printed in the United States of America 10 9 8 7 6 5

Human Kinetics
Web site: http://www.humankinetics.com/

United States: Human Kinetics, P.O. Box 5076, Champaign, IL 61825-5076
1-800-747-4457
e-mail: humank@hkusa.com

Canada: Human Kinetics, 475 Devonshire Road, Unit 100, Windsor, ON N8Y 2L5
1-800-465-7301 (in Canada only)
e-mail: humank@hkcanada.com

Europe: Human Kinetics, P.O. Box IW14, Leeds LS16 6TR, United Kingdom
+44 (0)113-278 1708
e-mail: humank@hkeurope.com

Australia: Human Kinetics, 57A Price Avenue, Lower Mitcham, South Australia 5062
(08) 82771555
e-mail: humank@hkaustralia.com

New Zealand: Human Kinetics, P.O. Box 105-231, Auckland Central
09-523-3462
e-mail: humank@hknewz.com

This book is dedicated to the only thing that really matters in life—family: Bev, Steve, Sue, Ben, James, Beau, Luann, Max, and Rachel.

Contents

Preface

Between the two of us, we have devoted more than 50 years of our lives to fitness and training for sports. We've been fortunate to have worked with thousands of athletes ranging from peewee sport participants and weekend warriors to elite amateurs and professionals. Each of these individuals has had specific objectives on which their training was focused. These are some of the more common concerns they have expressed:

- How can I improve my vertical jump?
- I need to be faster.
- I get knocked off-balance easily.
- I need to improve the accuracy of my tennis stroke.
- How can I develop greater power in my batting swing?
- I like to jog, but my low back gets sore.
- When I'm playing racquetball, I have trouble changing directions.

We typically respond to these and similar questions by advising people to develop a very important but often neglected part of the body: the abdominals and low back. This region is often referred to as the "center of power," trunk and low torso, or simply, "the core."

The abdominals are a major link in the body's musculoskeletal chain, yet they are typically the weak link. For thousands of years, athletes have been aware of the value of a strong core. You rarely see an ancient Greek sculpture of an athlete with a pot belly. Martial arts emphasize the importance of the "Ki," which means energy; and the "Hara," which indicates the physical center of the body. When Ki is focused in the Hara you become "centered" and have access to limitless energy. So it's not surprising that the center of power has become a primary concept in most modern conditioning programs. In fact, we place such value on the center of power that its training is the number one emphasis of our day-to-day conditioning regimen.

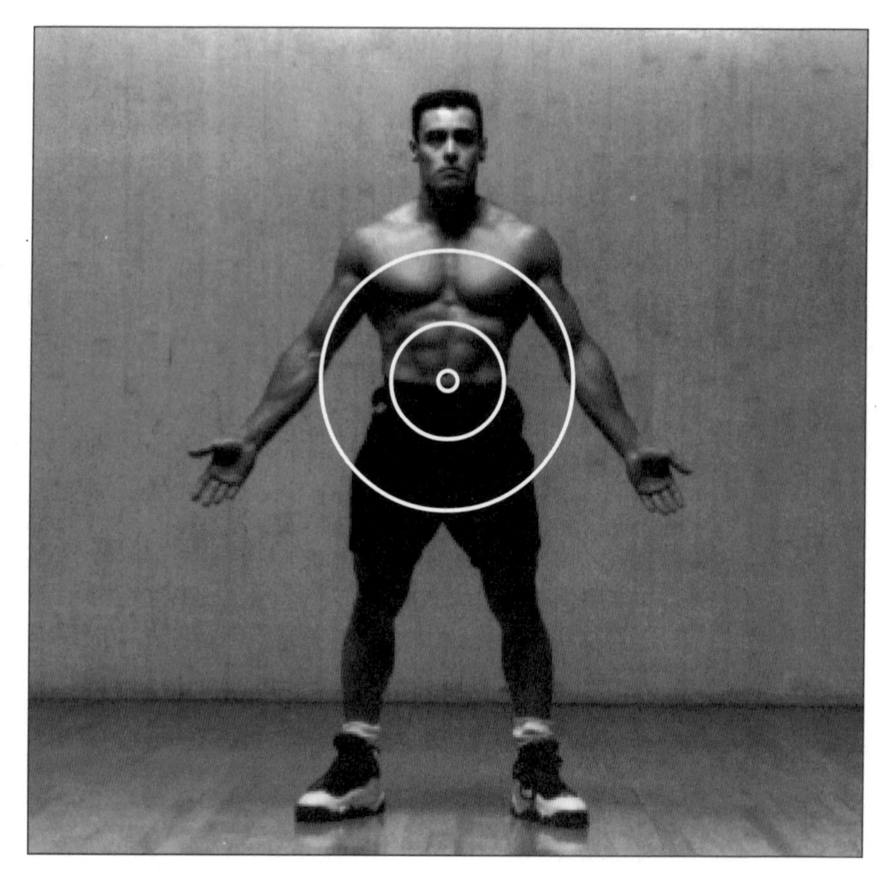

All of the teams and athletes we currently work with (such as the New York Knicks and four 1996 Olympians) underscore the importance of a regular habit of training the center of power. Consider the following facts:

- The trunk and low torso, which is the power center of the body, constitutes over 50 percent of your body's total mass.
- The muscles of the lower torso are essential for maintaining the body's equilibrium when performing most physical tasks.
- In addition to assisting efficient and proper movement, the abdominals help protect vital organs.
- The abdominals provide internal (intra-abdominal) pressure that supports the spine, maintaining the stability necessary to stand erect while decreasing low back stress.
- Core muscles also assist in breathing during exercise and sport performance.

Poorly developed abs do little to provide an anchor for explosive sports movements, much less general fitness. We cannot overemphasize the importance of developing and maintaining the center of power. In this book we have intentionally excluded other important variables relating to health, fitness, and total athletic development, focusing exclusively on the core. This does not mean, of course, that you should neglect other aspects of fitness. For example, in working with the Knicks, we never sacrifice other factors of athleticism, such as power, speed, quickness, flexibility, agility, coordination, endurance conditioning, mental toughness, and nutrition for an extra 10 minutes of ab work. Nor should you ignore other critical components of health and fitness, such as muscular strength, muscular endurance, cardiorespiratory efficiency, flexibility, and body composition. But since the center of power is the core from which all other athletic and fitness variables originate, concentrating on this area will enhance any athletic or fitness program.

In this book we will show you—whether you're an athlete or a fitness enthusiast—exactly how to train your center of power, which is the first step to developing total body power, speed, quickness, agility, coordination, or just a great set of abs. As you read, concentrate on *your* needs, whether you wish to improve sports performance or maintain a healthy lifestyle. While we refer often to the athlete, all of the training principles we discuss apply to the general fitness enthusiast as well.

The exercises illustrated in chapters 6, 7, and 8 are divided into three categories as follows:

Chapter 6	**Fitness:**	Fitness enthusiasts and all athletes
Chapter 7	**Strength:**	Advanced fitness enthusiasts and intermediate to advanced athletes
Chapter 8	**Power:**	Advanced athletes

Note: At this point and throughout the book, we will regularly emphasize that advancement to the power category carries risks. These drills are strictly for the experienced athlete. They should not be the goal of the fitness enthusiast. In fact, many elite level athletes are perfectly content to train with the fitness and strength drills, only incorporating the power drills if there is a specific need.

This organization enables you to tailor a program to *your* needs. Whatever your motivation, whether to dunk a basketball, add 10 yards to your golf drive, run a marathon, perform household chores without fear of injury, or simply look and feel better, you will benefit from this program.

This is not another book making the hollow promise that "If you follow this program, you'll have washboard abs in two weeks." If your motivation extends beyond vanity into the realm of improving fitness, maintaining health, or enhancing athletic performance, this book is for you. No shortcuts to developing your center of power exist, but if you stay with this program, adopting it as part of a disciplined lifestyle, you will see significant results. The regimen works, but—like any other program—is only as good as the consistent effort you put into it and your commitment to improvement.

Acknowledgments

To our remarkably patient editor, Elaine Mustain, whose great advice and incessantly positive attitude eased the arduous and often tedious publishing process, and ultimately made this book a reality. To Dr. John Ozmun of Indiana State University and Dr. Alan Mikesky of Indiana University Medical Center for their reliability, competence, and literary assistance. To Dr. Clifford Colwell of Scripps Clinic for his support, vision, and belief in our program. To Mark McKown, Director of Sports Performance at the College of Charleston, a leader in the strength and conditioning profession, for his friendship, insights, and persistent encouragement.

Thanks to our incredibly tolerant models John Starks, Charlie Ward, Kristin Denehy, and Michael Panetta for their voluntary involvement with the many days of grueling abdominal and low back exercise demonstration; and to John Sann, our photographer, who did an outstanding job of accurately capturing the essence of each drill though subjected to the limitation of using only one photo per drill.

To many mentors, coaches, teams, and athletes from all levels of development and all areas of the world who have touched our lives and made a difference in cultivating our perpetually expanding philosophy. To name a few: Pat Riley, Raymond Berry, Jeff Van Gundy, Tom Osborne, Patrick Ewing, Dale Murphy, Hal Morris, Steve Finley, Pam Shriver, Todd Martin, Jim Courier, Mary Joe Fernandez, Zach Thomas, Irving Fryer, New York Knicks, Orlando Magic, Indiana Pacers, Baltimore Orioles, Chicago Cubs, University of Nebraska, University of Colorado, Notre Dame University, Indiana University, Denver Broncos, Minnesota Vikings, Kansas City Chiefs, New Orleans Saints, New England Patriots, U.S.A. Olympic Cycling, U.S.A. Olympic Bobsled, U.S. Tennis Association, and U.S. Gymnastics Federation.

And finally, to Steve Brittenham, whose genius and pioneering insights in the field of developmental athleticism are matched only by his unceasing efforts to help children and aspiring young athletes *enjoy* the sports experience. He is an inspiration to all who have had the good fortune to work with him. Although professional athletes could certainly benefit from his considerable expertise, the future champions of the sports world have gained immeasurably through his continued contributions.

1

A Strong Core for Sports Performance

All force generated by upper- and lower-body musculature either originates, is stabilized by, or is transferred through the trunk and low torso. The body's center of gravity, an imaginary point around which the body's weight is evenly distributed, is also located in the low torso.

THE IMPORTANCE OF THE CORE

The maturation of movement skills begins with the core musculature and extends outward from that point. The formal term for this process is *proximal-to-distal development. Motor development* (movement skill) begins with the larger and slower muscles of the core (proximal muscles) early in a child's life. As a healthy child matures, development moves out gradually from the gross motor patterns of the core to the fine motor skills, which are controlled by the smallest muscles of the extremities (distal muscles). Whether you perform a fine motor skill, such as throwing darts, or a gross motor pattern, such as lifting a baby from a crib, you must have a strong core to ensure efficient and effective function.

Stability of Movement

The location of your center of gravity is important for stability. The exact location of this point will vary among individuals and will also change depending on the activity involved. For example, when a pole vaulter is "piking" over the bar, the center of gravity can actually be located outside the body (see figure on page 2). Since you can move this point simply by changing your position, you can make critical adjustments in your own stability.

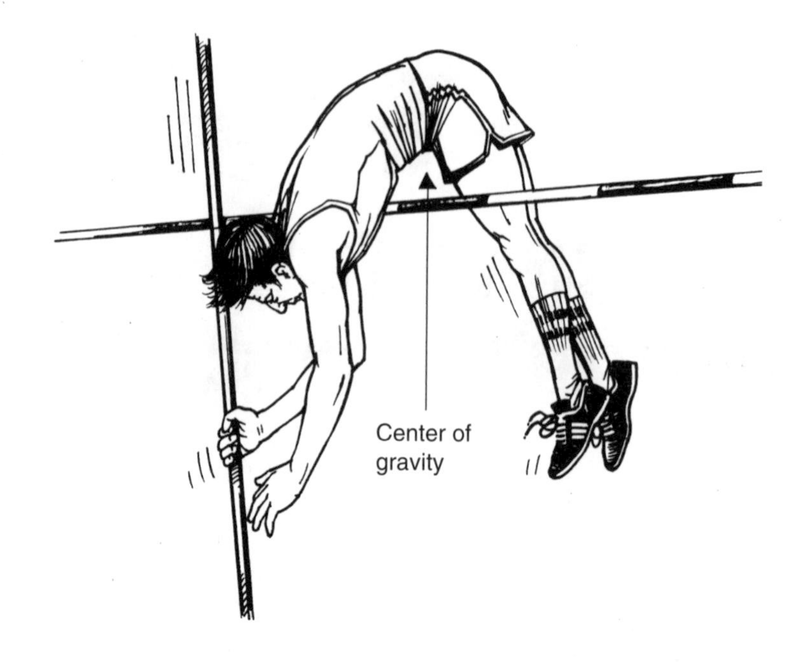

Two important ways in which you can adjust your stability are widening your base of support and lowering your center of gravity. For example, a wrestler can increase stability and decrease vulnerability if he assumes a wide stance, maintaining a low center of gravity by flexing his ankles, knees, and hips (see photo on page 3). And what makes a karate punch so powerful? It is thrown from a stable position. Yet, even though your center of gravity will continually shift—depending on the activity you're involved in—it typically remains at, or close to, a position approximately two inches below your navel (an important reason why an effective defender often focuses on the opponent's navel).

Transfer of Power

When you stand erect, your center of gravity is also the midpoint of your center of power. Successful athletic movements, or even simple household chores like working in the garden, can be enhanced simply by understanding the relationship between the center of gravity and the intended movement. Developing your center of power will greatly improve the efficiency and effectiveness of your physical actions. I'm sure you have heard the old saying, "A chain is only as strong as its weakest link." For the vast majority of people, the weak link in the body is the center of power. Let's look at an example.

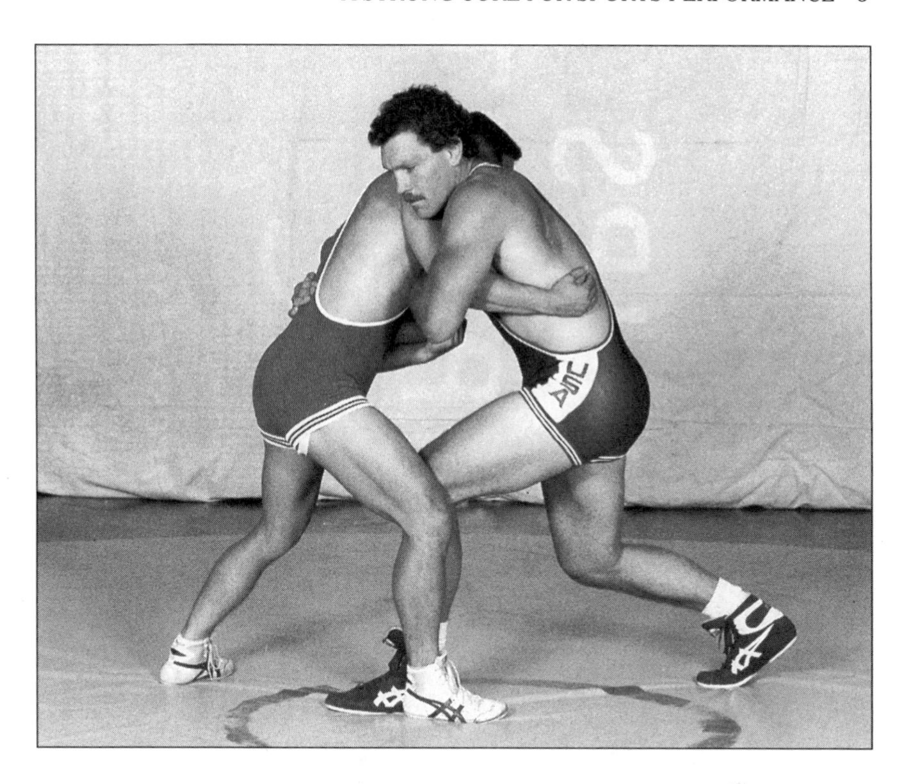

Imagine that a pencil represents your legs, and—to your credit—you have the strongest legs in the world. You have spent hundreds of hours training your legs. Unfortunately, you have neglected to train your trunk and low torso: Imagine that a Jell-O cube represents your torso. Your basketball coach has requested that you jump up and touch the rim, 10 feet above the floor—a task that shouldn't pose a challenge, given your incredible leg strength. But when you attempt to jump using your powerful legs, what happens to the Jell-O cube? (See figure *a* on page 4.)

Six months later, having developed your abs and low back, you have a strong core, represented by the rock. Now when you're asked to use your strong legs to perform an explosive task, such as touching the rim, you achieve tremendous results. (See figure *b* on page 4.) No matter how much force you exert against the rock with your legs, there will be nearly a 100 percent transfer of power through the rock to the upper body.

This "coupling" action created by a strong core connects movements of the lower body to the upper body and vice versa. In the example, when the force you generate by the triple extension of your

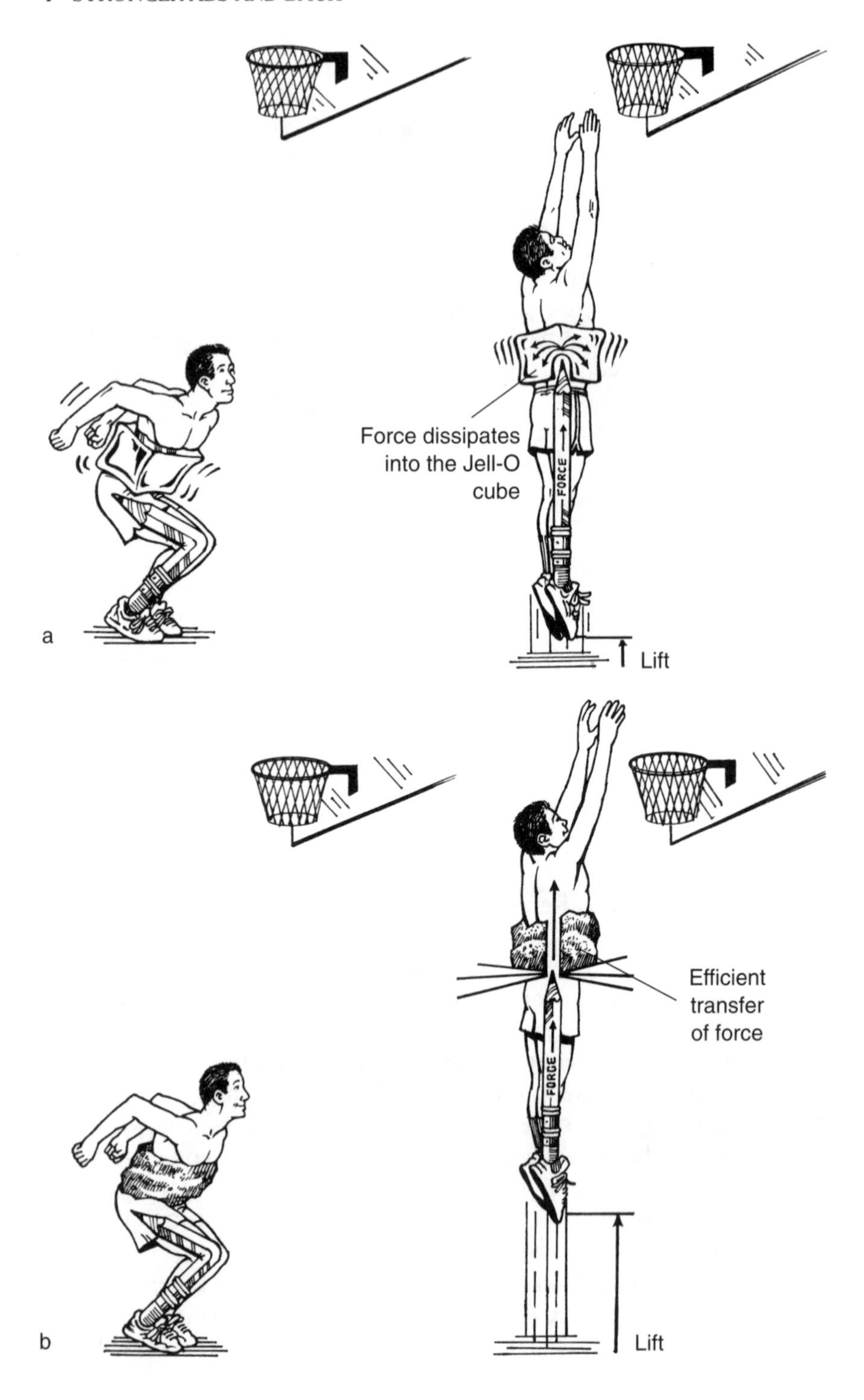
Force dissipates into the Jell-O cube
FORCE
Lift
a
Efficient transfer of force
FORCE
Lift
b

ankle, knee, and hip joints transfers through a solid area, little energy dissipates, giving you both greater power potential and more efficient movement. In short, the abdominals, the foundation on which all explosive movements are based, are no longer the weak link in the chain. Think in terms of increased power transfer when throwing, striking, jumping, running, mowing the lawn, picking up a heavy box, and the like. By eliminating your Jell-O cube, you are, in effect, creating the potential to utilize a greater percentage of upper and lower body musculature to perform a task. This means more efficient, accurate, and powerful movements. Not a bad tradeoff for devoting a modest portion of your total training program to the development of your center of power.

Efficiency of Action

So what role does the center of power play in movements that involve specific limbs, such as kicking, striking, or throwing? Regulating the torso requires delicate neural control and an efficient muscular system. The best tennis forehands and backhands, golf and baseball swings, slap shots, fast balls, curve balls, and extra point kicks are all controlled by the center of power. A well-developed core inhibits unnecessary movements. For example, if the goal of a sprinter is to run straight ahead, then she should channel all of her energy toward that goal. Arms that swing from side to side across the body or knees that flare to the sides detract from the goal of sprinting straight ahead. The great athlete conserves energy because her finely tuned core gives her the ability to make every motion effective, enabling her to move efficiently for longer periods.

Body Alignment

Offsetting the often detrimental effects of gravity is the key to an outstanding sports performance. One way to do this is to strive for proper body alignment. Force is transferred most efficiently through the body in a straight line, but because of poorly developed centers of power, athletes often have poor posture, which can lead to less efficient movements (see figure on page 6). Such athletes will not be able to maximize their power potentials, often wasting energy through jerky, uncoordinated, and extraneous movements. Moreover, because they lack the abdominal strength to maintain proper body alignment, they are prime candidates for injury.

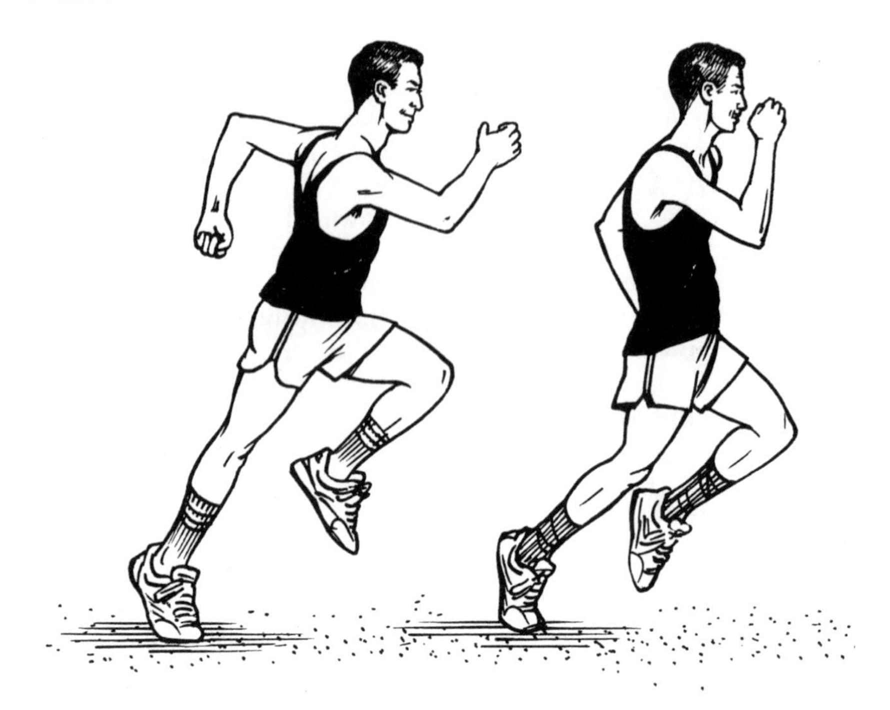

DEVELOPING THE CORE AND TRAINING FOR STRENGTH

Muscular strength is defined as the ability of a muscle or group of muscles to exert force maximally in one effort. *Muscular endurance* is the ability of a muscle or group of muscles to exert force repeatedly over an extended period of time. Developing both muscular strength and muscular endurance is of paramount concern for most serious athletes. In sport, with most factors being equal between two competitors, the stronger athlete will more than likely win. Likewise, strength is a fundamental ingredient in the fitness formula. The most obvious benefits of strength training include

- improved muscular strength,
- improved muscular endurance,
- improved power,
- improved motor control (athleticism), and
- decreased risk of injury.

Two Philosophies of Strength Training

A misguided yet popular philosophy of strength training for athletes persists: Focus training mainly on the region of the body most obviously needed to succeed in the sport. For example, if the sport places major emphasis on pushing, throwing, and pulling, then strength training of the upper body is generally the major concern. This is followed by a lower body routine and finally—if time permits—the center of power region. If the sport requires jumping, sprinting, or kicking, training typically focuses on the lower body, followed by the upper body, and finally—if time—the center of power region. In order to develop an athlete's full strength and power potential, the primary focus of the training program should be the abdominals and low back—given the fact that all movements either originate in or are *coupled* through the core—followed by the development of those principal muscles specific to the actions or movements unique to the sport.

Progressive Overload

The history of strength training extends far back to a time when athletic success often equaled the death of the opponent. Not wanting to suffer such a fate, a Greek wrestler, Milo of Crotona, devised what was probably the first progressive resistance training program. Legend has it that each day Milo would lift a cow across his shoulders and walk across a stadium. He began when the cow was a young calf and continued his program, carrying the same animal until it reached adulthood (see figure on page 8). Naturally, each day as the cow grew older and heavier, Milo was required to adapt to the increased resistance by a matching increase in strength. For 24 years, Milo was undefeated in the wrestling arena.

Primitive as it was, we still use Milo's concept of progressive overload today when we increase the stress we place on a muscle as it becomes capable of producing greater force.

Absolute Versus Relative Strength

Unfortunately, most coaches, athletes, and fitness enthusiasts measure the success of their strength training program by absolute strength, or the maximum amount of force that a muscle or group of muscles can generate. To determine a more accurate measure of progress, however, assess your strength-to-weight ratio, or relative

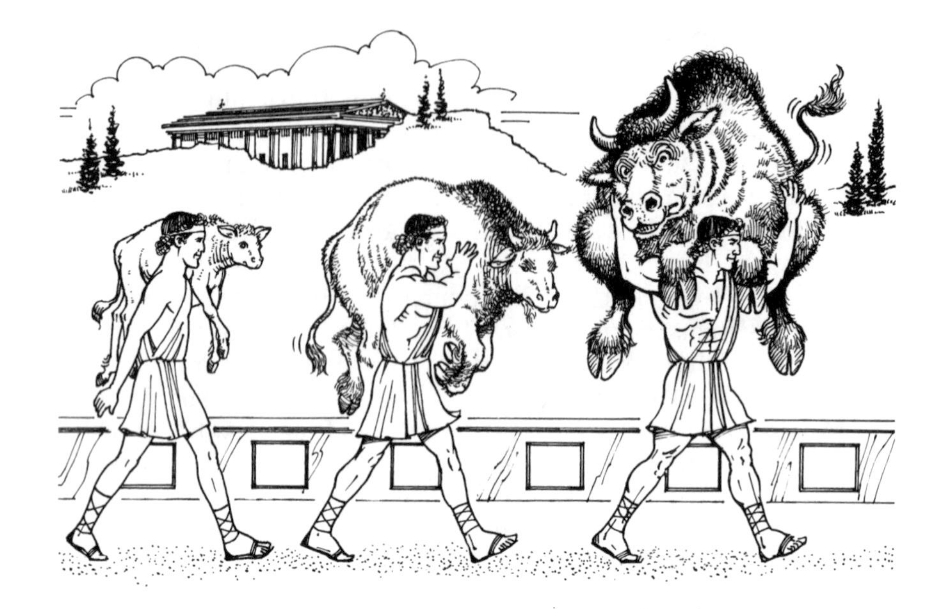

strength. Relative strength is expressed as strength per pound of body weight. In this way, we can more accurately make a strength comparison between two individuals of differing body types. For example, a person who weighs 150 pounds successfully lifts 250 pounds while a person who weighs 250 pounds is capable of lifting 350 pounds. The heavier person has, of course, greater absolute strength but the lighter person has greater relative strength. He has lifted more weight per pound of body weight (about 1.7 pounds) than the larger person (1.4 pounds).

Dynamic Training

The muscles of the trunk and torso are responsible not only for the maintenance of posture, but also for the necessary efficiency of movement associated with all athletic activities. The trunk and torso are capable of movements throughout a limitless number of planes. Therefore, static, one-plane strength training is not very practical. The dynamic nature of sport dictates that, for a strength program to be effective, you must develop the center of power to work the way you need it to. Activities incorporating flexion, extension, rotation, and the infinite number of combinations of these three basic movements will more fully develop the core. All athletic movements and activities of daily life depend on this dynamic foundation. Fortify this essential link and ensure the effectiveness of your entire training regimen. You'll not only develop your abs, you'll strengthen your entire body.

Establishing Goals

Athlete or not, it is important to establish training goals. Whether your aim is to increase the velocity of your tennis stroke or to add three inches to your vertical jump, determine which muscles are involved in the movement or action and design a program that specifically and progressively stresses those muscles. Include specific training activities that closely mimic the motor patterns, muscle involvement, and speeds encountered during the actual activity or athletic event. Then, gradually and safely build upon your skills. To help you, we've included a wide variety of trunk and torso exercises in this manual that you can perform at different velocities and angles. Assess the demands of your sport or activity, determine the involvement of the abdominal and low back musculature, and then emphasize the exercises that meet the demands.

Myths About Strength Training

Many people believe that strength training will make them muscle-bound, slow, tight, or heavy; or that muscle will turn into fat once they stop training. The majority of these ideas are completely unfounded. Strength training can actually enhance flexibility when performed correctly through a full range of motion. If you are concerned about putting on weight, understand that a greater potential for force production exists when you increase the size and therefore the weight of your muscles. For example, 10 additional pounds of muscle mass can move a lot more than just 10 pounds. Furthermore, even if you were to stop strength training for an extended period of time, your muscle fibers may lose some size, but it is physiologically impossible for muscle tissue to change into fat. The major reason that athletes who decrease training tend to see an increase in fat is that although they no longer need to consume the large quantities of food necessary to fuel high-level training, they often continue to eat the same high-calorie diet, causing the excess calories to be redirected into fat.

DEVELOPING THE CORE AND TRAINING FOR POWER

Acquiring strength is just one component of developing your center of power. Sports movements typically require explosive, ballistic, and well-coordinated muscular actions. The ability to take strength that is gained from the weight room and apply it effectively on the playing field is the ultimate goal of any strength training program. The strongest athlete is not necessarily the most powerful athlete. Power and strength are not synonymous. Power is dependent on strength and speed, thus the term "speed strength." In order for athletes to maximize their power gains, they must include a *speed* component in their training.

$$\text{Power} = (\text{Force} \times \text{Distance})/\text{Time}$$

Simply put, power is a relationship between strength and speed.

Speed can be defined as the time it takes to move from point *A* to point *B*. The distance between point *A* and point *B* could be the 26.2 miles of a marathon, the 10 feet from the floor to the basketball rim, or, when at bat, from the "cocked" position to the contact point with the ball. Once you combine speed with strength, the long hours in the weight room start to pay off, and sport-specific or *functional* strength translates to power.

Say, for example, two athletes are performing a bench press. Both are attempting to lift the same weight. The first athlete lowers the bar to his chest, then pushes the weight up to a straight arm position. The time required to move the bar from point *A* (the chest) to point *B* (the locked arm position) took three seconds. With the second athlete, the elapsed time to move the bar from point *A* to point *B* was only one second. The weight lifted by both athletes was identical, but the shorter time by the second lifter indicates greater power output.

The athlete who labors to build muscular strength should also integrate speed equally into the training program. Linking the power components of speed and strength will lead to excellence in sports performance.

Developing Speed

Developing the speed component of power differs dramatically from standard programs designed to enhance strength. Typically, you can increase your muscular strength through consistent and progressive training with weights. Training for speed, however, is not as easily accomplished through regular trips to the weight room. Factors pertaining to speed development include

1. individual genetic characteristics, and
2. the physiology of the muscular system.

Individual Genetic Characteristics and Their Relationship to Speed

Muscle fiber types (i.e., muscle cell types) influence speed. For our purposes, we'll discuss two types of muscle fiber, fast-twitch and slow-twitch. The fast-twitch fibers exert great power, but they fatigue quickly. The body generates the energy required to contract a fast-twitch fiber anaerobically, or without oxygen. These fibers are better suited for short, explosive actions, such as sprints, Olympic lifting, and volleyball spikes. In contrast, the slow-twitch fibers require oxygen for sustained contraction and, therefore, are ideal for endurance activities, such as cross-country skiing, marathon running, or bicycle racing in the Tour de France. Athletes who participate in endurance sports typically have a higher percentage of slow-twitch fibers in the muscles that are predominately in use for those sports. Conversely, the muscles of athletes whose sports require explosive actions tend to contain a higher percentage of fast-twitch fibers. Most elite level athletes gravitate toward sports that are compatible with their genetic makeup.

All of us were born with a certain ratio of fast-twitch to slow-twitch fibers. Even if your muscles are predominantly slow-twitch, however, it does not necessarily mean you are destined to remain slow. Granted, you will never be as fast as a cheetah, but you can always become faster than you are right now. You simply must learn how to maximize what you have inherited.

One way to do this is by using a greater percentage of your fast-twitch capability. Here's an example (assume both athletes are the same height and weight):

Athlete one has 52 percent fast-twitch muscle fibers and 48 percent slow-twitch muscle fibers.

Athlete two has 48 percent fast-twitch muscle fibers and 52 percent slow-twitch muscle fibers.

Both athletes are tested in the vertical jump, which is a good way to measure leg power:

Athlete one (predominately fast-twitch) jumps 24 inches.

Athlete two (predominately slow-twitch) jumps 26 inches.

How can this be? Athlete one, given his genetics, should out-jump athlete two. If we could determine what percentage of muscle was used to perform the task, we might see that athlete one used 75 percent of his fast-twitch potential while athlete two used 85 percent of his.

Athlete one: 52 percent genetic fast × 75 percent utilization = 39 percent of potential.

Athlete two: 48 percent genetic fast × 85 percent utilization = 41 percent of potential.

Therefore, no matter what people might say or what you might think about "being slow," no one has reached his potential, and each of us has tremendous room for improvement. Training can either enhance or partially overcome genetics.

Muscle Physiology and Its Impact on Speed

One way to tap into your vast reservoir of potential is to further develop your naturally occurring physiological processes.

Stretch Reflex. For example, the speed component of power is directly influenced by a highly trainable attribute referred to as the *stretch reflex*. If you were to examine a muscle through a microscope, you would discover tiny sensory mechanisms called muscle spindles. These spindles are about the size of a muscle fiber (or cell) and are located among, and parallel to, the muscle fibers (see figure below). A spindle's primary responsibility is to prevent injury to the fibers in

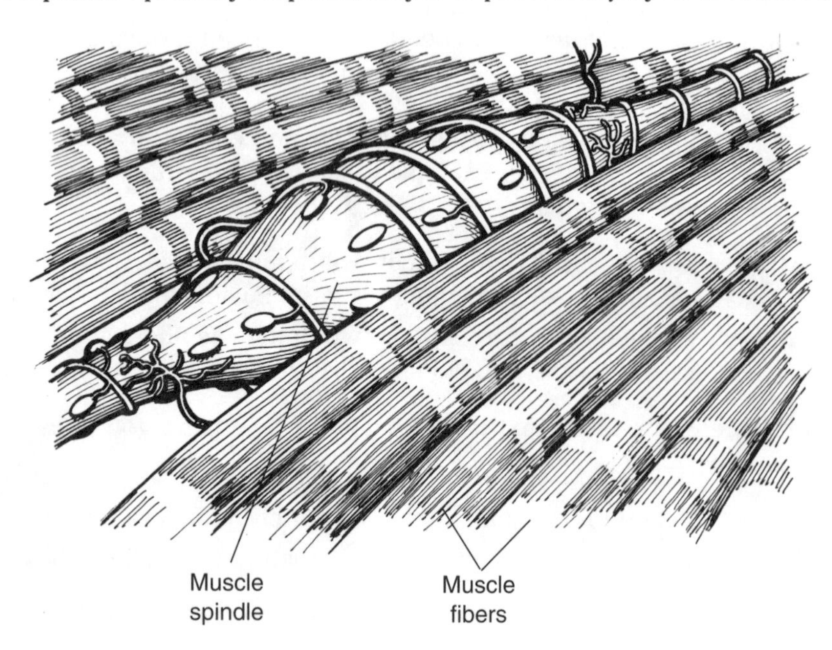

situations where the fibers might be placed on an excessively rapid and/or overly forceful stretch beyond the muscle's tolerance, which can certainly occur due to the ballistic nature of most athletic movements. The muscles, however, can also use the spindles to generate a more powerful contraction. Here's how it works. In the photos below, the athlete is performing a vertical jump (sometimes referred to as a "countermovement" jump).

The jump places those muscles that span the shoulder, hip, knee, and ankle on a *rapid stretch,* primarily as a result of gravity and body weight. Since the muscle spindles lie parallel to the muscle fibers, they, too, undergo a stretch. The spindles sense the stretch and send a message to the central nervous system (brain and spinal cord). In turn, the central nervous system instructs the stretched muscles to contract more forcefully, depending on the speed and magnitude of the stretch. If this sensory mechanism did not exist, or for some reason was not functioning, the rapid stretch would most certainly cause

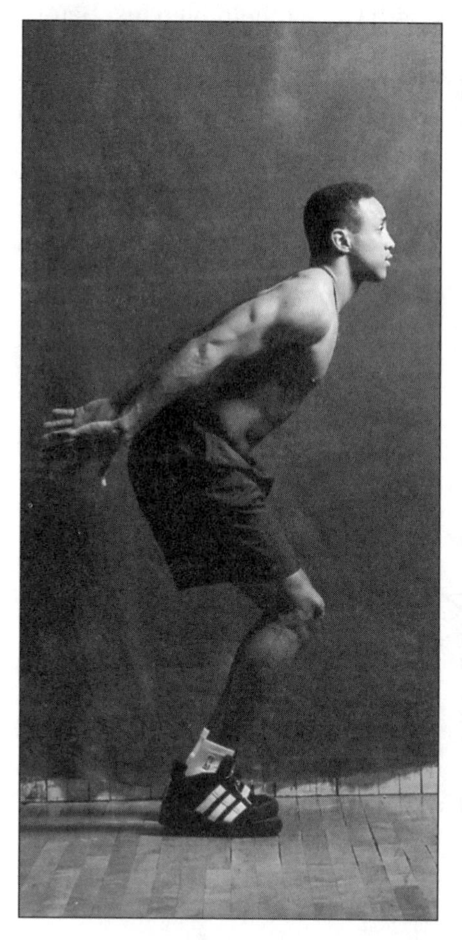

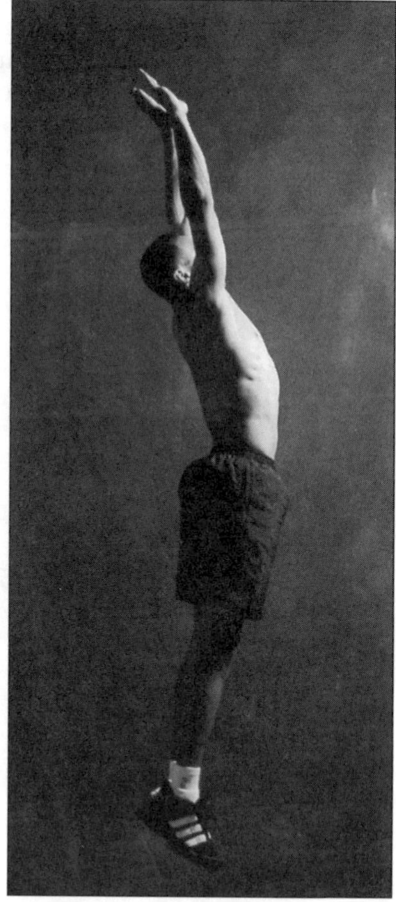

an injury to the muscle. The muscle spindle response, when combined with a subsequent voluntary, or intended, contraction, can help the athlete perform more explosive movements.

Stored Elastic Energy. Another important physiological phenomenon of muscle is called *stored elastic energy.* Think of a rubber band stretching. Imagine that the elasticity of the rubber is similar to the elastic properties of a muscle (fibers) and its tendon. As you stretch the rubber band, you store energy in the elastic properties of the rubber. When you release one end, you release that stored energy (see figure below). An important difference exists, however, between a rubber band and muscle fiber. With the rubber band, the longer the stretch, the more energy is stored and then released. But with muscle fiber, it's not the magnitude, but rather the speed, of the stretch that determines how much energy is stored for use during the immediate ensuing contraction.

You can take advantage of the inherent elasticity of muscle. The baseball batter "cocking" the body with the bat held high just before swinging or the discus thrower "snapping" (rotating the hips) just prior to throwing are prime examples of this *stretch-shortening cycle.* This physiological process is definitely trainable, and most progres-

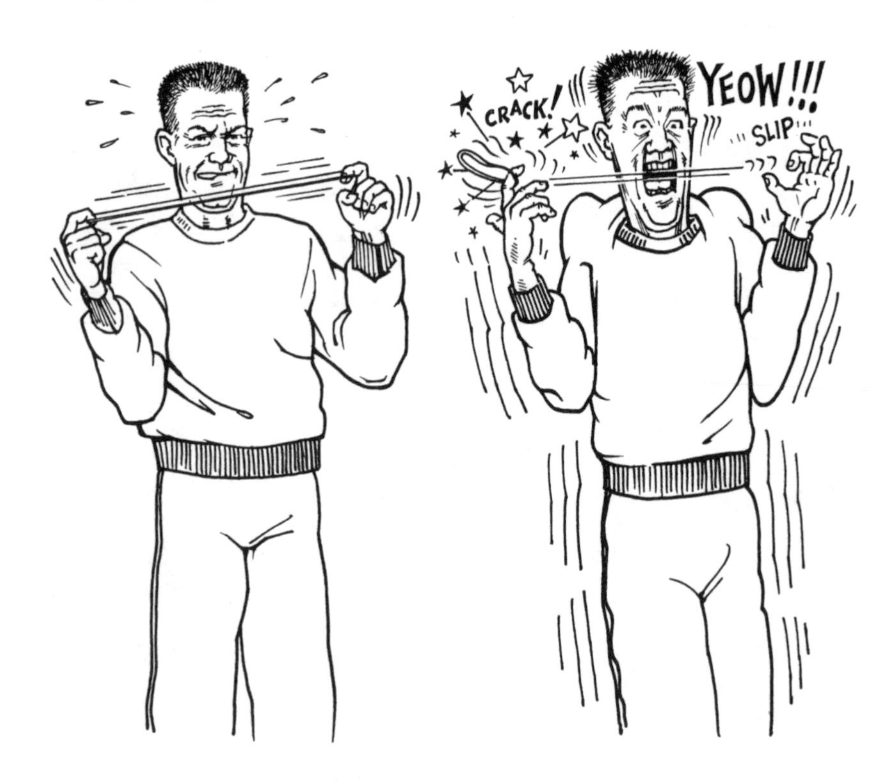

sive regimens employ drills and activities designed to enhance these processes.

To a lesser extent, the stretch-shortening cycle can help you recruit a greater percentage of muscle to perform a given task. Consequently, your power potential will be more thoroughly exploited. Superior power in the core region will directly enhance all athletic movements. The technical term for this mode of training incorporating the muscle spindle and muscle elasticity is *plyometrics*. Several of the exercises we will outline in chapter 8 specifically address the training of the stretch-shortening cycle of the abdominals through the use of plyometrics.

Why some athletes have successfully scratched the surface of their physical potential a little deeper than the rest of us will always remain a mystery. But remember, no matter what your current ability, you can improve.

DEVELOPING AGILITY

With a clearer understanding of the importance of strength and speed, you can begin to tap into your vast reservoir of dormant potential. Be aware, however, that possessing speed and strength is one thing; the ability to control and use it on the playing field is quite another. Fortunately, for sports requiring rapid changes of direction such as basketball, racquetball, tennis, and volleyball, a well-developed center of power will greatly enhance your agility. Agility is closely related to stability and is the ability to change direction accurately without sacrificing speed. This is sometimes referred to as *dynamic balance*. Many athletes are cut from teams not because they lack the necessary speed, but because they cannot effectively control the speed they have.

Akin to agility, stability, and dynamic balance is *automaticity* (sometimes referred to as kinesthetic sense). Have you ever noticed how some athletes have an uncanny ability to "see" the entire playing floor, knowing just when to deliver the basketball to a teammate for an easy layup? Or have you watched a tennis player who is at the net when her opponent hits a lob and who, without watching the ball, sprints to the back of the court and turns so that the ball drops right at her feet, setting up the perfect forehand smash? This is sometimes referred to as "court sense" and is a quality that we all possess—in varying degrees.

Great athletes seem to have "eyes in the back of their heads" when it comes to performing spectacular moves to the basket or delivering the football the split second an opening appears. This ability has also been referred to as the "zone of relaxed concentration." Jerry Rice, Steffi Graff, Anfernee Hardaway, Greg Maddux, and Michael Jordan are prime examples of athletes who regularly perform in this zone. Automaticity is knowing what the muscles are doing in relation to the environment. This *spatial awareness* is a "feel" for one's immediate surroundings. Feeling smooth or awkward, effortless or forced, in balance or out of control stimulates continual feedback, resulting in necessary adjustments.

The ability to achieve maximum results with minimum effort indicates a highly refined kinesthetic awareness. As you experiment with many of the exercises in this manual, you will notice that the bilateral (i.e., works both sides of the body) nature of the exercises are very similar to actual sport skills. Assess the specific skills required to perform your sport, then choose those exercises that most closely mimic those skills, and emphasize developing the center of power muscles specific to your movement and skill needs.

2

A Strong Core for Fitness

So far we've focused on center of power development for athletic performance. But a strong core is equally critical for general health and fitness. For example, low back pain is one of the most common ailments among adults in the United States. Approximately 80 percent of the population will, at some point, endure low back problems. Low back pain accounts for more lost hours from work than any other occupational injury. Chronic low back pain afflicts millions of people each day. Insurance companies spend millions on the treatment of low back pain resulting from injuries that could have been prevented. Even athletes are not immune to the debilitating effects of low back pain. In 1995, 38% of all professional tennis players missed at least one tournament because of a back problem.

THE ANATOMY OF YOUR BACK

Your spine is a complicated structure and, together with the sternum and ribs, constitutes the skeletal foundation of the body's trunk and torso. In a healthy adult spine, 26 vertebrae run from the base of the skull down to the rear pelvis.

The vertebral column encases the fragile spinal cord, providing vital protection. Aided by the muscles of the core, the spine supports the head, helps maintain erect posture, and facilitates a multitude of movements, including bending and twisting. In between each vertebrae are *intervertebral discs*. The discs are composed of a tough outer *fibrocartilage* ring filled with a soft, jelly-like substance. These discs compress, allowing for movement and acting as shock absorbers.

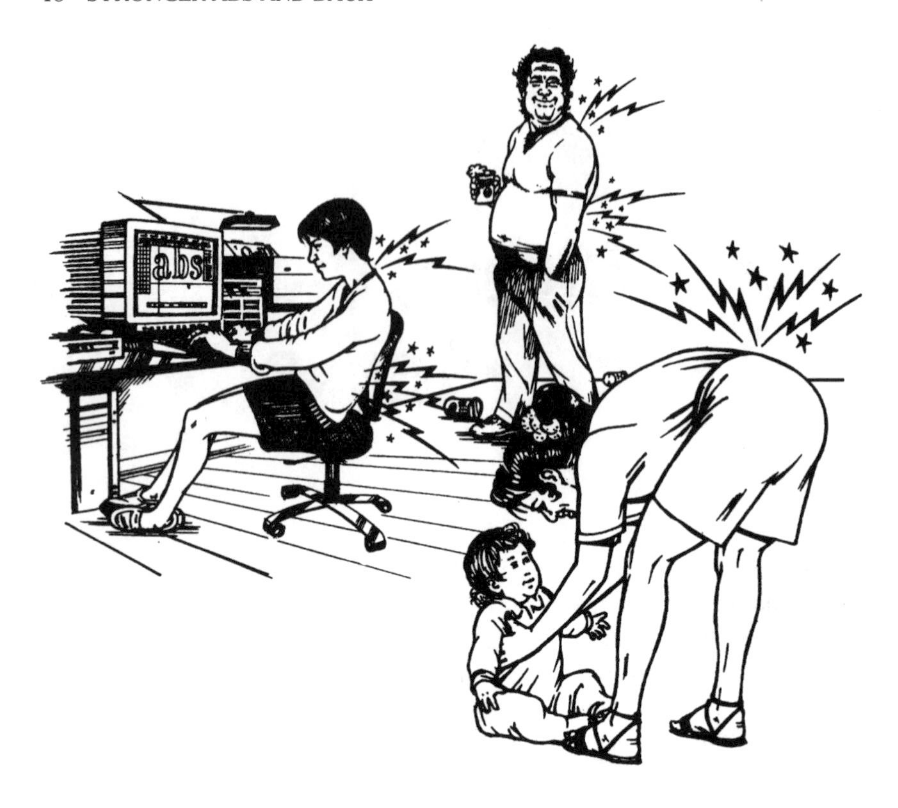

Unfortunately, we tend to abuse this intricate structure through poor lifting habits; poor posture while standing, sitting, sleeping, or walking; and generally being out of shape.

A STRONG CORE AND BACK PAIN

What is the exact cause of low back pain? No one is sure, but lack of flexibility, poor posture, obesity, stress and tension, and inactivity are all potential contributors to low back problems. Muscular factors including weaknesses and strength imbalances are often directly or indirectly the culprits.

Support of the Spine

A weak trunk and torso can lead to extraneous movements. In turn, inefficient movement, particularly while a person is fatigued, can be a primary source of injury. Strong back muscles increase the stability of the spine and prevent excessive stress on supportive structures, such as ligaments and the connective tissue surrounding the discs. Strong abdominal muscles contribute to the support of the spine by increasing internal pressure in much the same way that a lifting belt supports the weight lifter during a heavy workout. This increased intra-abdominal pressure helps relieve the load on the spinal discs.

Alignment of the Pelvis

Pelvic alignment is also influenced by the muscles of the lower torso. An extreme forward (anterior) or backward (posterior) pelvic tilt has been linked to low back pain. Two sets of opposing (antagonist) muscles combine to maintain the structural integrity of the pelvic region. The hip flexors tilt the pelvis forward while the hip extensors and abdominal muscles tilt the pelvis backward. Lack of strength or flexibility in either or both of these areas can lead to poor alignment and, ultimately, to back pain. Having adequate strength to perform daily tasks such as picking up a baby, raking leaves, or sitting at your computer for long hours is key to reducing the frequency and severity of low back pain.

Low Back Pain Prevention

To help avoid low back pain, follow these preventative measures:

1. Before initiating any new exercise routine consult your physician. If you are recovering from a back or abdominal injury, be sure your doctor or trainer approves *all* exercises you wish to include in your center of power training regimen.
2. Occasionally, doctors misdiagnose the cause of low back pain or dismiss it as a sign of stress or fatigue. Therefore, if pain persists, consult a back specialist. A doctor or therapist can prescribe treatments for structural deviations, such as swayback, scoliosis, or leg length discrepancies.
3. Strengthen the supportive muscles of the core region. This book will help!
4. Always prepare your body for physical activity. Include stretching exercises during both warm-up and cooldown. Emphasize those muscles that are prone to excessive tightness. (See chapter 3, "Warm-Up, Stretching, and Cooldown.")

5. Always use your legs to lift heavy objects: keep knees flexed, back straight, and body close to the object.

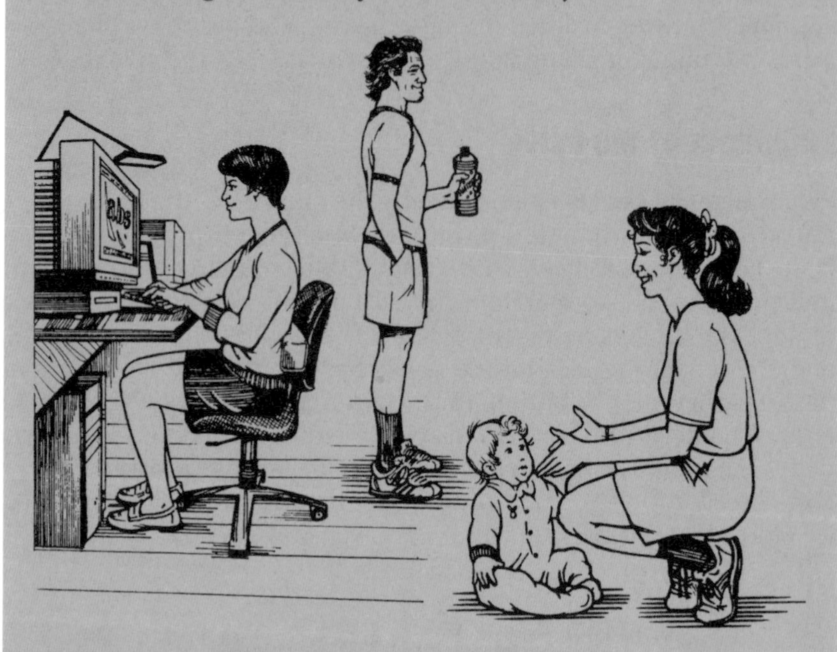

6. Try to lose excess weight, especially from your midsection. This can cause forward pelvic tilt, leading to lower back tension.
7. Avoid exercises that place undue stress on the low back, such as straight-leg sit-ups. Also, several drills in this book are geared toward the seasoned professional. No one who has been diagnosed as a candidate for low back pain, or who already suffers from it, should attempt the more demanding, sports-oriented exercises in this manual.
8. Most importantly, practice good posture at all times.

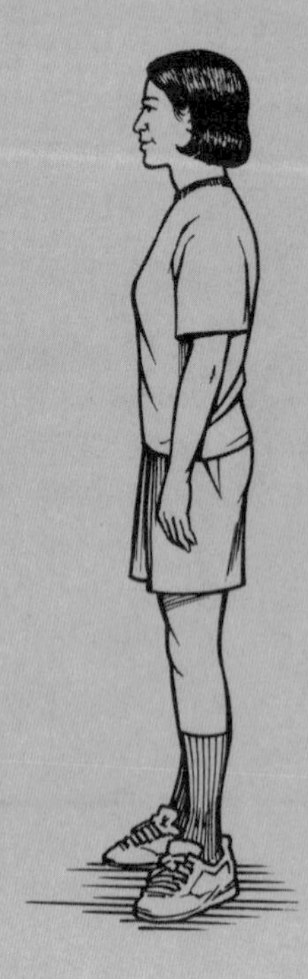

SYNERGISTIC TRAINING

The low back and torso are capable of many movements. All the muscles of the center of power work together to perform these many functions. However, you can isolate muscular regions of the trunk and torso and thereby develop strength and power in a specific movement. If we train each *part* of the center of power from a variety of angles and with challenging methods, the *whole* becomes more powerful. This is the concept of *synergy*.

Knowing that the muscles of the abdominal region are interdependent, we have designed a training program that will stress the weaker supportive muscles first, and then will focus on the stronger action muscles as the program progresses. This is important for surviving the workout and using the time most efficiently without becoming too tired to practice correct technique.

The center of power region includes some of the largest muscles in the body. Adhering to the concept of synergy, all the muscles of the trunk and torso must be equally and progressively challenged to enhance efficient functioning. Likewise, a wide variety of movements must be incorporated to ensure total development.

Abdominal Muscles

The primary muscles of the abdominal wall are pictured in the figure on page 22.

Working together, these muscles can flex the spine forward and sideways, rotate the lower and upper body, and compress the abdomen, which, as noted earlier, is important for creating the internal pressure supporting the low back. Moreover, the ability to control abdominal pressure will assist in diaphragm breathing techniques. The *transversus* is a particularly important muscle to women who have experienced pregnancy and childbirth. Want to recapture your flat, prepregnancy belly? Work on the transversus!

Back Muscles

Like the abdominals, the muscles of the back are critically important to the proper functioning of the spine and therefore of the center of power.

The muscles illustrated in the figure on page 23 help maintain low back integrity. Superficial back muscles, which lie over the *spinalis* group, also contribute to the stability and action of the low back and upper torso. These include the *trapezius*, *rhomboids*, *latissimus dorsi*, and *serratus* group. The muscles of the buttocks and legs stabilize the

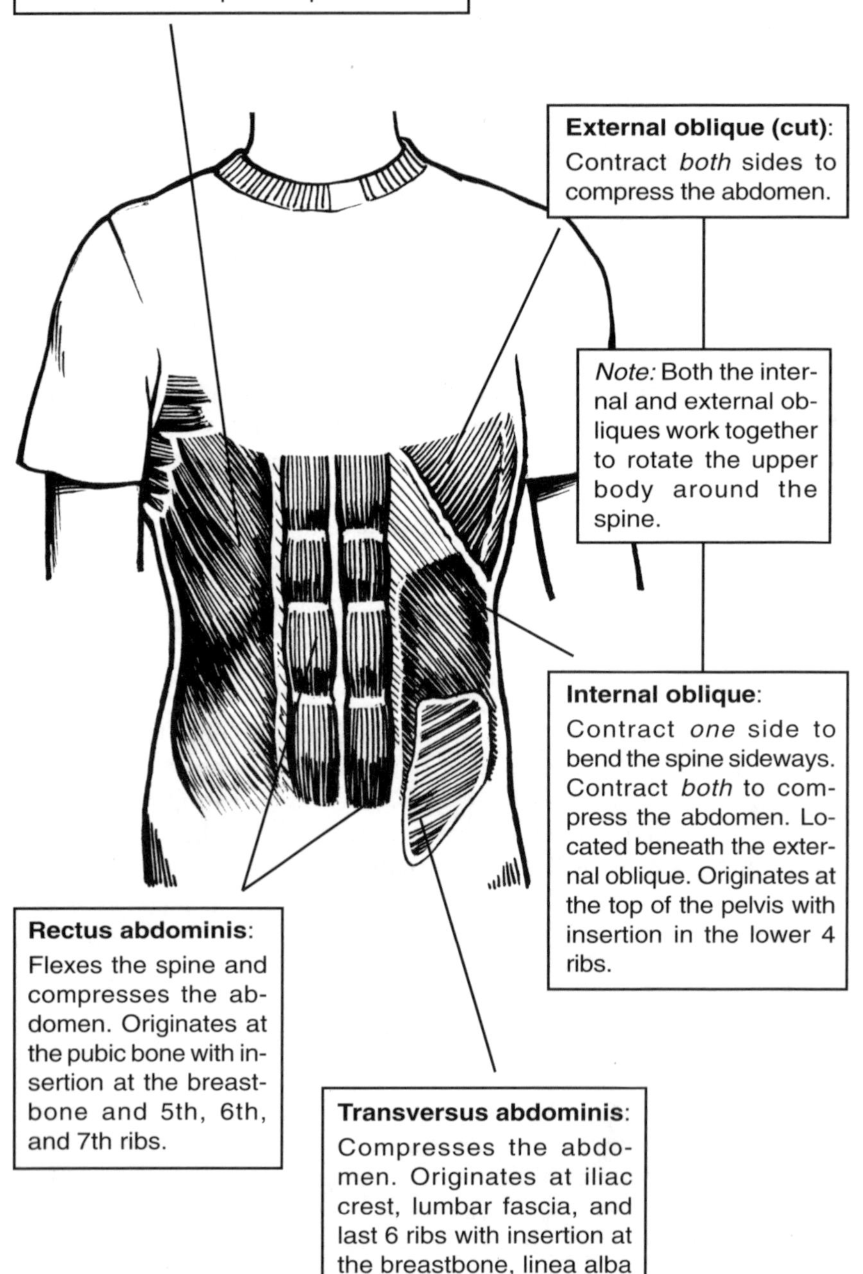
External oblique:
Contract *one* side to bend the spine sideways. Originates in lower 8 ribs with insertion at the top of the pelvis.
External oblique (cut):
Contract *both* sides to compress the abdomen.
Note: Both the internal and external obliques work together to rotate the upper body around the spine.
Internal oblique:
Contract *one* side to bend the spine sideways. Contract *both* to compress the abdomen. Located beneath the external oblique. Originates at the top of the pelvis with insertion in the lower 4 ribs.
Rectus abdominis:
Flexes the spine and compresses the abdomen. Originates at the pubic bone with insertion at the breastbone and 5th, 6th, and 7th ribs.
Transversus abdominis:
Compresses the abdomen. Originates at iliac crest, lumbar fascia, and last 6 ribs with insertion at the breastbone, linea alba to pubic bone.

Spinalis group:
Extends the spine. This muscle group runs the entire length of the vertebral column; however, the main mass is located in the lumbar region.

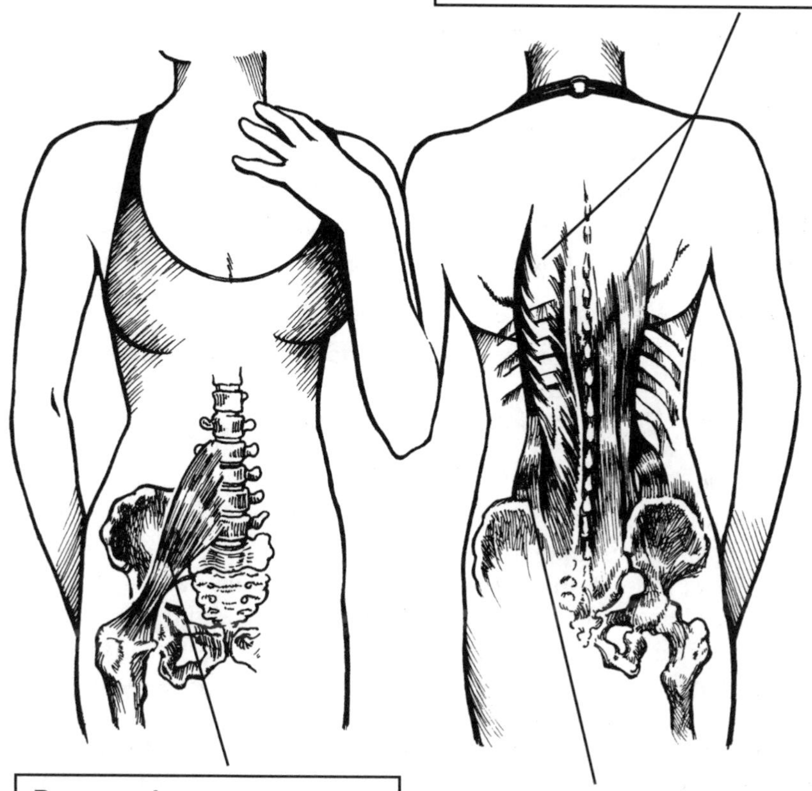

Psoas major:
Flexes and rotates the thigh sideways and flexes the spine. Originates at the lower 6 vertebrae with insertion at the femur (front of the leg).

Quadratus lumborum:
Flexes the spine sideways. Originates at the top of the pelvis with insertion at the 12th rib and upper 4 lumbar vertebrae.

Note: Psoas major is primarily a hip flexor, but since it also flexes the spine it has been included in the low back muscles.

pelvis and control pelvic rotation. The extensors and flexors of the hip are directly involved in movements of the low trunk, specifically the *gluteus maximus* and hamstrings. To create a total training approach to developing your center of power, incorporate exercises that stress this supporting musculature.

Identifying the Focus of Each Exercise

To keep matters simple, we will refer to the center of power musculature through their *regional* identities, not by their anatomical names. Each exercise is associated with a particular movement or the development of a specific region of the trunk and low torso. With some drill modification, you can shift the emphasis from one region to another. The regions include the following:

Obliques	Internal and external obliques
Lower abs	Lower portion, rectus abdominis, and transversus abdominis
Upper abs	Upper portion, rectus abdominis
Back	All low back musculature

Identifying an exercise with a particular region doesn't mean that other musculature outside the region are not involved. Quite the contrary. For example, if an exercise identifies the lower abs as the primary mover, the supporting muscles of the trunk and low torso will act as stabilizers. They may even help in the lift, especially as the primary mover becomes fatigued. We will discuss this in detail in chapter 4, "Training Guidelines."

If you're aiming for a strictly abdominal workout, isolate your abs by limiting the range of motion to less than 45 degrees from the floor (see photo on page 25). If you incorporate movement beyond 45 degrees, the strong thigh muscles (i.e., psoas and hip flexors) take over as the primary movers. Although the hip flexor muscles are used heavily in sports, and should therefore receive some attention, they should not be the main focus of an abdominal training session.

APPROACHING GREAT ABS: SETTING YOUR GOALS

So why do you want to improve your abs? Decide why, then create an abdominal training program tailored to your needs.

Do you want to rehabilitate your back, preventing or reducing pain? Do you want to improve your general health and fitness? Reduce weight? Gain weight? (Lucky you!) Achieve total body toning? Work

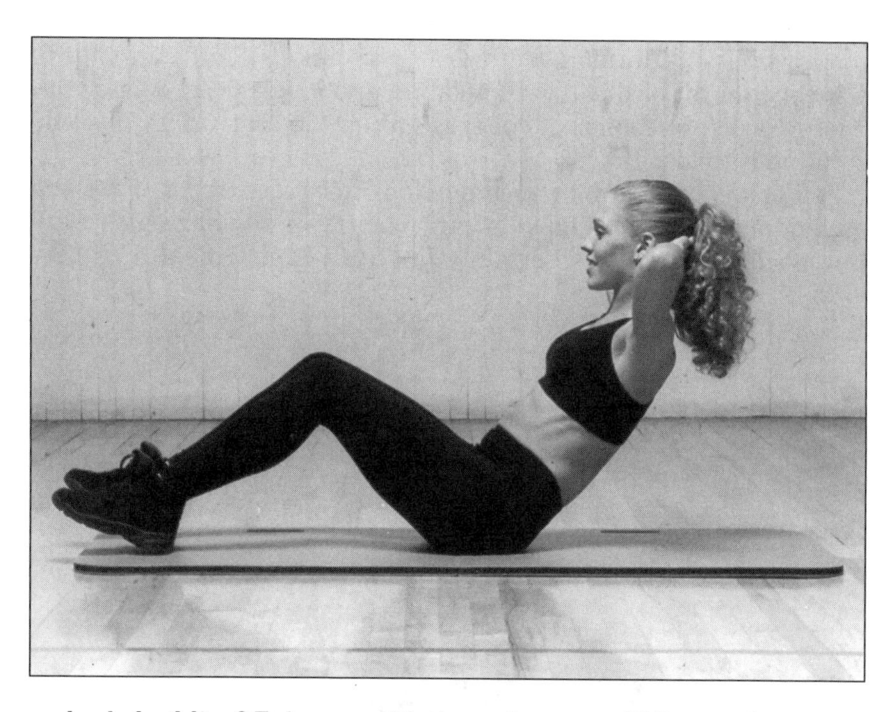

on body building? Enhance athletic performance? The combinations of motivations for beginning an exercise program are as varied as the readers who have purchased this book.

Set realistic goals. The "rippled" effect that is the pride and joy of all body builders is the result of a lifestyle committed to building mass. What we often see on the covers of those body building magazines is the end result of a precise combination of diet, endless hours in the weight room, and genetics. While the dream of washboard abs may be a great motivator, and while it may be achievable for some, for many others it is an unlikely goal. Decide what *you* want to achieve, remembering that, whatever your present physical condition, you can always improve.

Still, whatever your motivation, remember that while strengthening your core is critical to total body fitness, it is only the beginning of achieving complete physical fitness. Plan to build upon your newfound center of power to create a healthy overall structure.

THE SKINNY ON FAT REDUCTION

Are sit-ups enough? Not if a layer of fat blankets your abs. It's hard to see that "rippled" effect if the fat layer just below the skin is hiding your abs. You might know your abs are stronger, but no one else will until you lose the fat. Unfortunately, many misguided fitness enthusiasts toil for hours performing leg raises or sit-ups in a futile attempt to burn the fat off of these accumulation spots. But don't waste your energy on "spot reducing," because it just doesn't work. The only solution is to lose the fat.

Perhaps you are not interested in looking at a great set of abs and are adopting the program solely to alleviate or minimize the risk of low back pain. This is certainly fine, but from a health and fit-

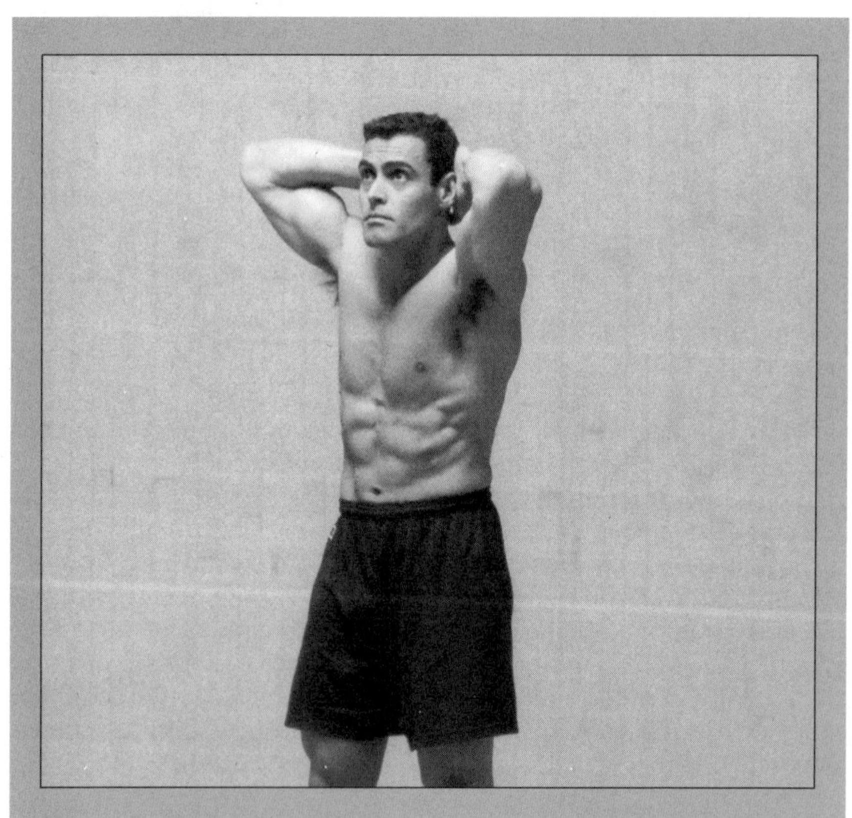

Interestingly, many times, particularly in some athletes, those "love handles," which congregate on your sides about waist level (just above the iliac crest), are not fat deposits but well-developed lower obliques. Performing additional oblique exercises to minimize the deceptive appearance of fat accumulation around the midsection may in fact create those very handles you're trying to eradicate. If your body fat levels are relatively low, and you still see those handles, place less emphasis on the oblique exercises. Athletes, however, should concentrate on equal and total core development. If the appearance of "muscle handles" are a by-product, you'll just have to learn to accept the fact.

ness perspective, it's still important that you don't let fat get out of hand.

Create a Caloric Deficit

The best way to lose excess fat is to create a caloric deficit whereby caloric expenditure (exercise) is greater than caloric intake (food consumption). To accomplish this, you have several options:

1. Reduce caloric intake.
2. Maintain present diet calories but increase caloric expenditure.
3. Both reduce intake and increase expenditure.

The combination approach makes the most sense because the reduction in food consumption it requires is less drastic than reducing caloric intake only, while the added exercise will improve your total caloric expenditure and overall health.

One pound of fat is equal to 3500 calories. During the course of one week, if you were to eliminate 500 calories per day from your diet, theoretically you could expect to lose one pound of fat per week. A 500-calorie *diet* reduction per day, however, could be very traumatic. A better approach is to exercise and burn away some of those 3500 calories. For example, if you expended 200 to 300 additional calories per day (see table 2.1), then you would require a diet deficit of only 200 to 300 calories—a more realistic amount. In one week you should lose one pound of fat.

What You Should Eat

You may expend more or fewer calories than someone else based on your level of activity. Likewise, you may eat more or less, depending on your eating habits. Athletes will require more calories than the normal population, but in general, no matter what your activity level or eating habits, you should receive about 60 to 70 percent of calories from carbohydrate, 10 to 15 percent from protein, and no more than 30 percent from fats, with less than 10 percent from saturated fats.

Avoid the allure of fad diets, monitor your fat and calorie intake, and make adjustments where necessary. If volume of food is important to you, keep in mind that one gram of carbohydrate or protein equals four calories, while one gram of fat equals nine calories. This means that you can eat twice as much carbohydrate or protein as fat and consume fewer calories. With correct information, it is possible to maintain a high energy, low calorie diet and lose a pound or two

TABLE 2.1 Summary of Energy Cost of Selected Physical Activities

Activity	Cal/min*
Bowling *(while active)*	7.0
Golfing *(foursome to twosome)*	3.7-5.0
Walking, road or field *(3.5 mph)*	5.6-7.0
Cycling *(easy to hard)*	5.0-15.0
Canoeing *(2.5 mph-4.0 mph)*	3.0-7.0
Swimming *(25-50 yd/min)*	6.0-12.5
Running *(10 min mile)*	12.5
Handball	10.0
Skipping rope	10.0-15.0
Running *(8 min mile)*	15.0
Running *(6 min mile)*	20.0

*Add 10% for each 15 lb over 150; subtract 10% for each 15 lb under 150.

Adapted, by permission, from B.J. Sharkey, 1997, *Fitness and health*, 4th ed. (Champaign, IL: Human Kinetics Publishers, Inc.), 239-241.

per week—a sensible goal for fat reduction. After a couple of months of exercise and a sensible diet, you'll notice positive trimming of your entire body.

Sticking to It

While the math is simple, the commitment is not. A great resource that can help you with motivation and solid information is *Nancy Clark's Sports Nutrition Guidebook* (2nd edition). Don't let the sports title discourage you. The information in this book is equally beneficial to the fitness enthusiast. Another strategy you can follow before taking any drastic steps with your diet is to contact the American Dietetic Association (216 West Jackson Boulevard, Chicago, IL, 60606-6995, 312-899-0040) or your physician for help in locating a registered dietitian or nutritional resources. Find the information and the support you need and stick to it!

3

Warm-Up, Stretching, and Cooldown

Before you jump right into your abdominal routine, remember that most injuries are the result of overworking a system that has not been adequately prepared for stress. It takes as little as 10 minutes to warm up and stretch your abs in preparation for physical work. The main purpose of a warm-up is to prepare the body for exercise and prevent injury to muscle and connective tissue (the noncontractile tendons that attach the muscle to the bone).

HOW TO WARM UP

Most warm-ups involve some sort of active movement, such as brisk walking, jogging, or calisthenics. As an athlete, you'll derive greater benefit if your warm-up closely mimics the actions central to your sport, position, or ensuing training activity. This prepares your motor skill coordinating system and heightens your kinesthetic awareness. A low intensity warm-up will stimulate the delivery of nutrients by the blood and increase enzyme activity in the working muscles. All this will result in improved accuracy, strength, speed, and muscle and tendon elasticity, which can decrease the chance of injury.

STRETCHING

The ability of a joint to move throughout its full range of motion, free of muscular or structural impingement, indicates flexibility. Everyone is different. Some are extremely "loose" and never have to work at their joint flexibility. Others are about as supple as a two-by-four. So how much flexibility should you strive for? If you're flexible enough to do easily whatever activities you need to do, you're OK, whether you're hanging clothes on the line or performing the splits on the balance beam.

Static or Dynamic?

The routines presented in this manual involve predominantly *static* stretches. For the developing athlete or the general population, a static routine can more than adequately stretch the trunk and low torso. Static stretching involves an initial slow movement of the muscle to a point of comfortable tension—you should not be in pain. Hold this position for at least 10 seconds—preferably 15 to 20. Be conscious of your limitations, avoiding stretching beyond the muscle's capability. Stretching is the best way to improve muscle pliability, thereby decreasing the frequency and severity of a soft tissue (muscle and tendon) injury. A flexibility routine involving strictly static stretches is all you'll need to prepare your trunk and torso for the exercises listed in chapters 6 and 7. *Dynamic* stretches require a greater kinesthetic awareness and knowledge of physical limitations than the average fitness enthusiast possesses. Therefore, we do not recommend them for the general population. Even an athlete, if unaccustomed to this form of stretching, is at a slight risk of injury. But given the nature of some of the more advanced power development exercises (chapter 8) and the often explosive characteristics of most sports movements, a dynamic routine would be warranted. Otherwise, stick to the static stretches.

How Much Warm-Up or Stretching Is Enough?

You should spend three to five minutes in some sort of low intensity activity, such as walking, calisthenics, or jogging. Then allow another five minutes or so to stretch the muscles you are about to work. Select six to eight stretches that address the entire core. Place greater emphasis on the tight areas of your body. If you intend to train the entire body, you'll need to spend additional time stretching.

Further Resources

Since the range of this manual is limited to developing the center of power, the following stretches will focus on that specific region of the body. From the standpoint of total fitness, however, we recommend that you use a flexibility routine that addresses all the major muscles of the body. If you want to know more about stretching, your local bookstore can provide books on everything from the proven, traditional Tai Chi methods to the contemporary (and quite effective) Active Isolated patterns emerging from the Sarasota, Florida clinic of flexibility guru Aaron Mattes.

THE COOLDOWN

Don't forget your cooldown—one of the most overlooked elements of any training program. The stretches that follow are an effective part of that phase of your program as well. While it is understandable that the last thing you want to do after a long strenuous workout is to spend an additional 5 to 10 minutes cooling down, it might be the most important 5 to 10 minutes of the entire workout.

During physical activity, your body is expending energy, muscle fibers "break down," core body temperature rises, heart rate accelerates, and a host of other physiological phenomena take place. If your body cannot adequately recover from all these stresses between workouts, a collapse will occur in the system, and you will stop making progress. But allowing sufficient recovery after you stress your system will increase your abilities to heights above pre-stress levels, which is what progressive physical training is all about. (See figures below and on page 32.)

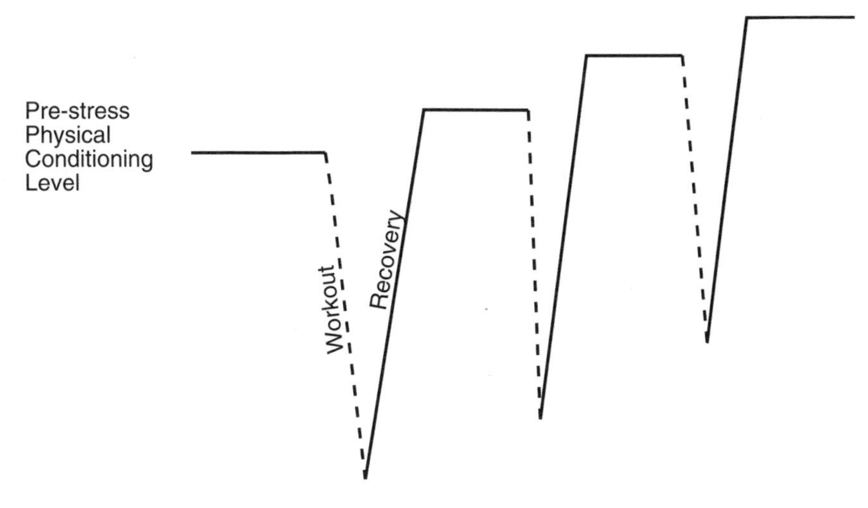

Positive Adaptation Effect

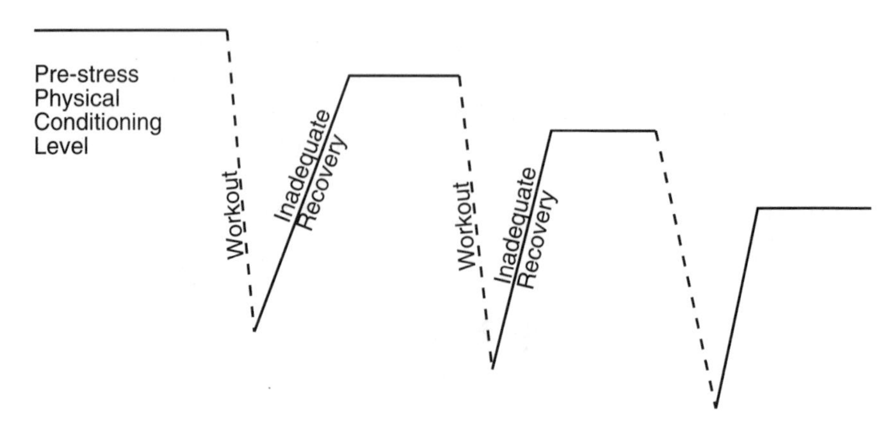

Negative Training Effect

A cooldown expedites the recovery process. A slow walk, jog, or calisthenics routine followed by static stretching assists in removing the leftover acids (the by-product of ATP synthesis) from the muscles, initiates the repairing of "micro" tears in the muscle fibers, facilitates the body's cooling system, and helps lower the heart rate to pre-stress levels, all of which prepares you for subsequent workouts.

Static Stretching Guidelines

- Never bounce or rapidly force a static stretch. Once you feel a comfortable tension, hold that position for a minimum of 10 seconds (preferably 15 to 20), then relax and repeat (several times if time allows).
- Keep your breathing slow and rhythmic. This helps your body relax, aiding in the stretching process.
- Study the examples, focusing your attention on correct technique, and try to isolate the muscles you're stretching.

Trunk and Low Torso Stretches

Standing Spinal Twist

Static: Standing

Stand 12 to 24 inches away from an opening (such as a power rack or doorway) with your back toward the opening. Reach back and grasp the rack or door frame. Gently twist to both sides of the body.

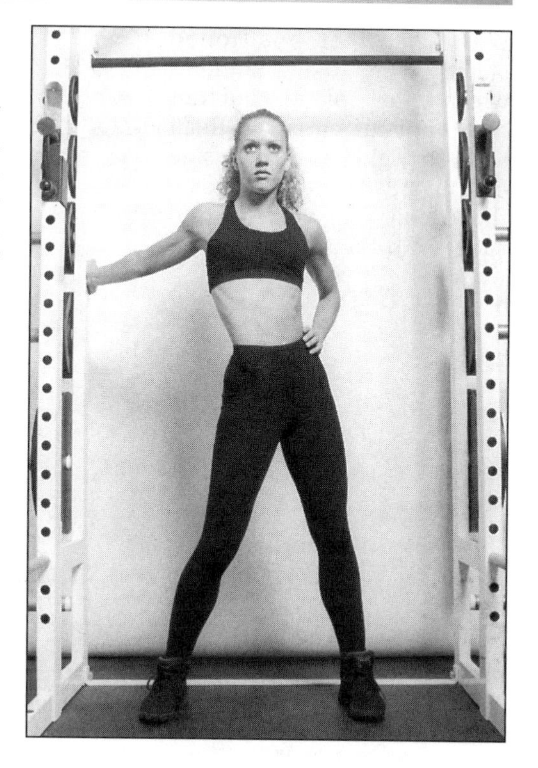

Low Back Press

Static: Standing

While standing with your feet together, slowly bend down and reach behind your bent knees. Lock your arms by clasping your elbows. Gently try to straighten your legs. Concentrate on "pushing up" through the low back. If performed correctly, your legs will never fully straighten.

Note: Avoid this stretch if you experience low back pain.

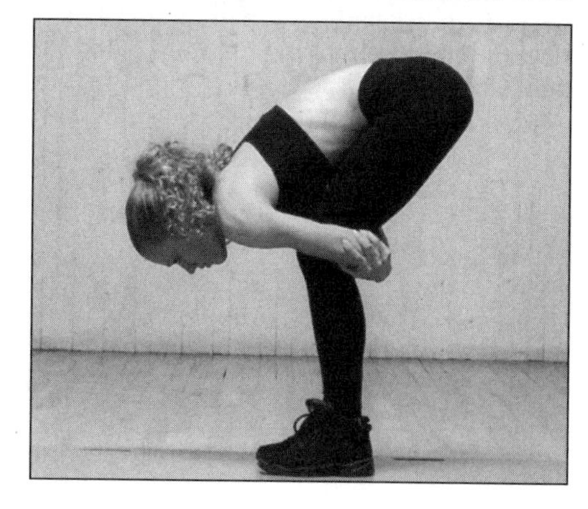

Side Bend

Static: Standing

With your feet positioned slightly wider than shoulder-width apart, place your left hand on your outer left thigh and your right hand on the side of your head. Slowly bend to the left, allowing your hand to slide down the leg. As always, work both sides.

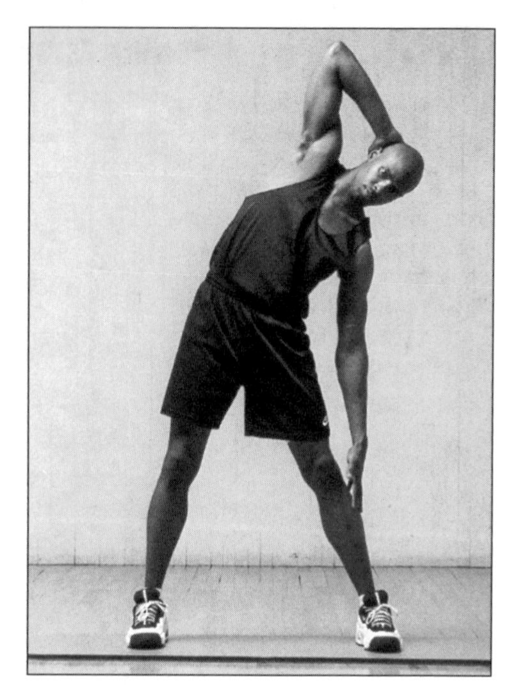

Seated Cat

Static: Floor

While sitting in a chair, slowly bend forward and grasp the chair's legs. Gently "push up" against the low back.

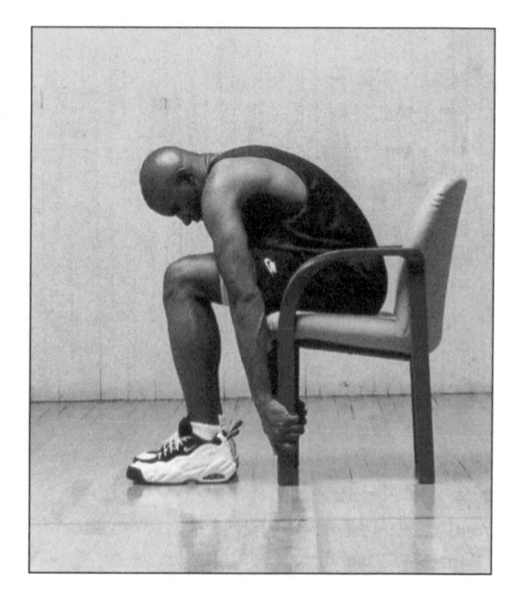

Mad Cat Arch

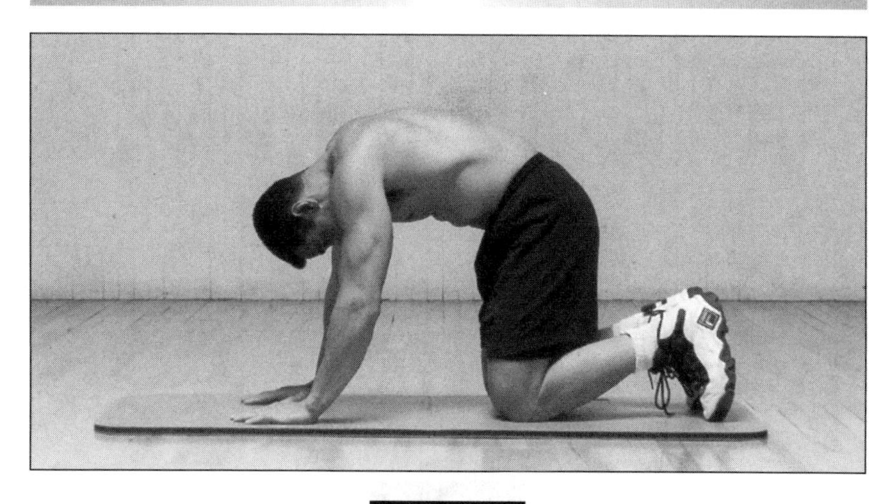

Static: Floor

On your hands and knees, tuck your chin and tighten your abdominals. Tilt your pelvis and lift, or "hunch" your back.

Mad Cat Leg Extension

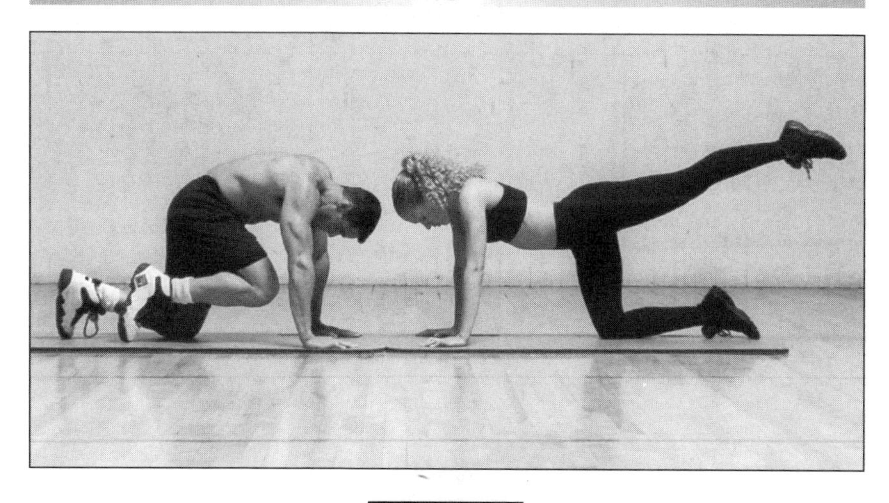

Static: Floor

From the hunched position of the Mad Cat Arch, tuck your right knee up toward your right shoulder. Then slowly extend the leg and lift your head, thus flattening your back. Remember to work both sides of your body.

Mad Cat Progression

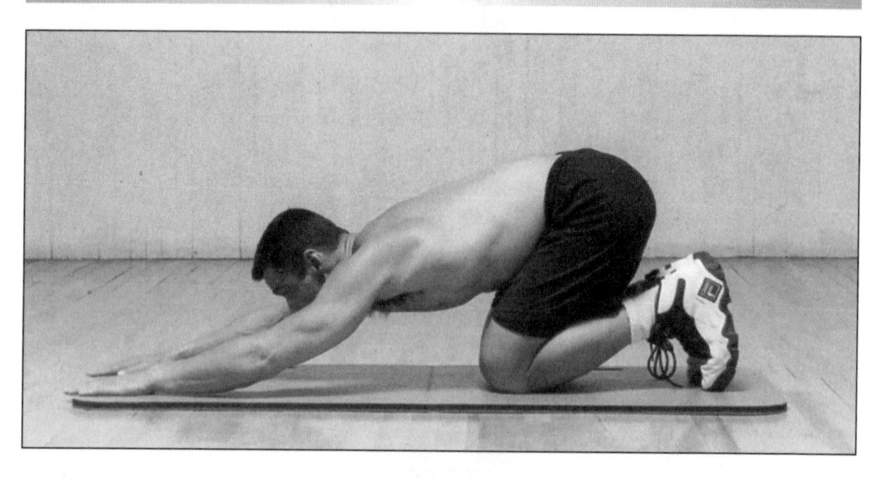

Static: Floor

While still kneeling, extend both arms overhead, keeping your hands flat on the floor. Lower your buttocks toward your heels. Slowly alternate pressure from your right side to your left.

Note: If you have some knee problems you may want to avoid this stretch.

Total Body

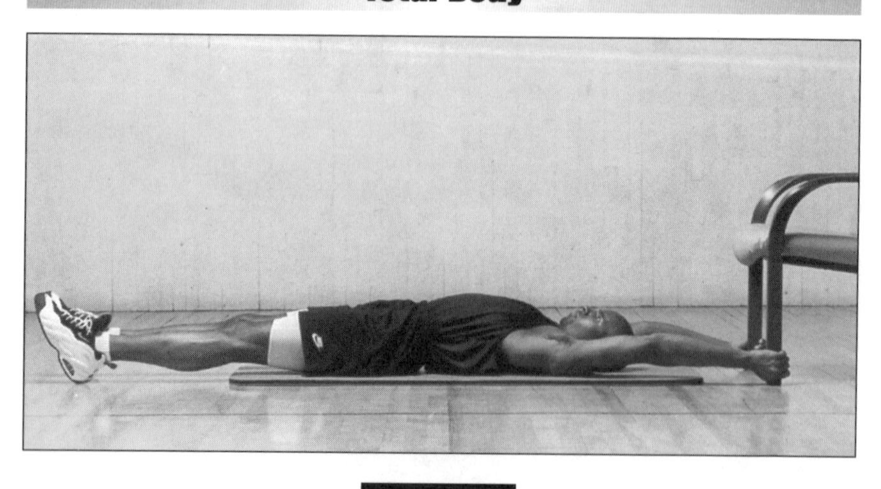

Static: Floor

Lie on your back with your arms and legs fully extended. Reach as far as possible in opposite directions.

Note: For a greater stretch, anchor your upper body by grabbing hold of a heavy or fixed object such as the legs of a sofa.

Crossed Leg

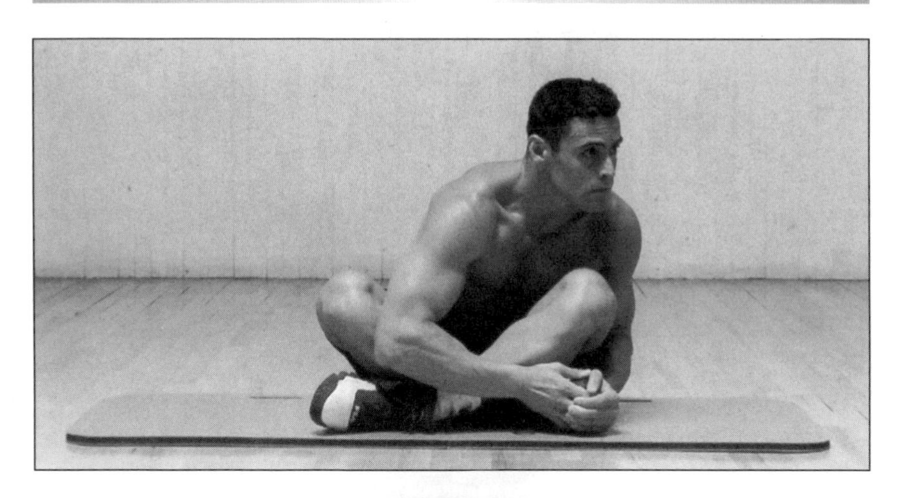

Static: Floor

While seated in a crossed-leg position, back straight and head up, lean out over the left knee, hold, then repeat with the right knee.

Seated Straight Leg

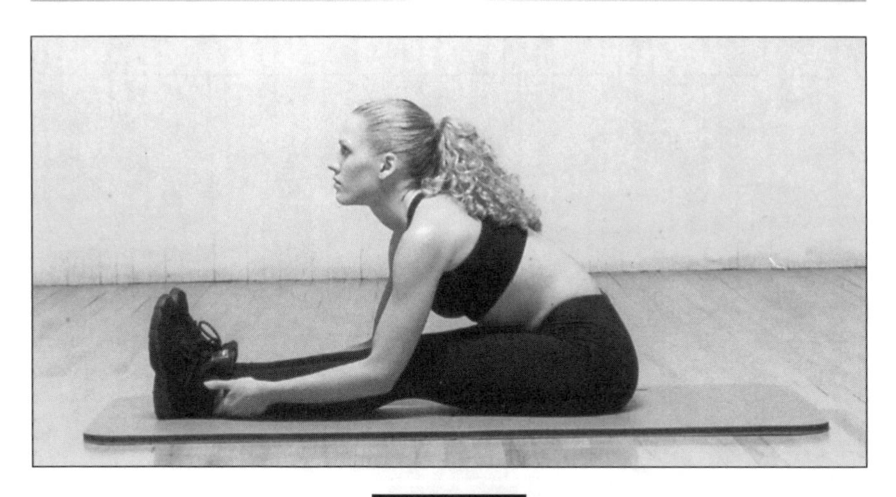

Static: Floor

This exercise mainly stretches the hamstrings, but for some tight individuals, it can be an excellent low back stretch. In a seated position with legs together and extended, back straight and head up, slowly lean forward until you feel a comfortable stretch. Remember to keep breathing.

Roll Back

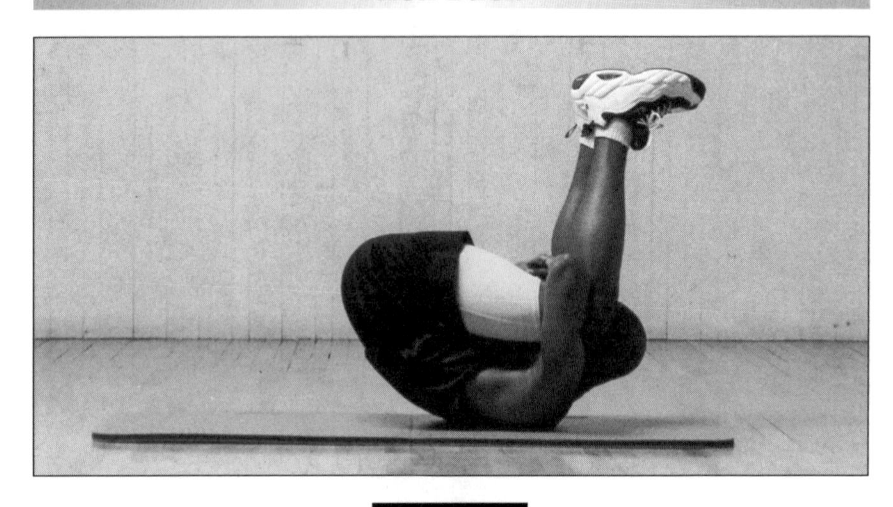

Static: Floor

While seated on a soft surface, arms clasped behind your knees, slowly roll back onto your shoulders. Keep your chin tucked to your chest and avoid rolling onto your neck. Rock back to the starting position and repeat.

Note: Avoid this exercise entirely if you have had any spinal problems.

Legs Spread

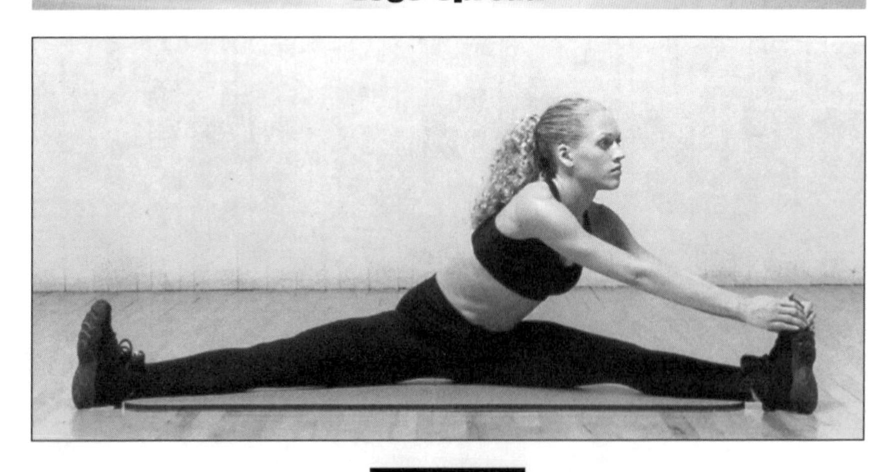

Static: Floor

In a seated position, spread your legs and point your toes toward the ceiling. With your back straight and head up, slowly exhale and reach toward your left foot, hold; repeat with the other foot. If necessary, place your hands on the floor to give you more support.

Legs Spread Progression: Side Stretch

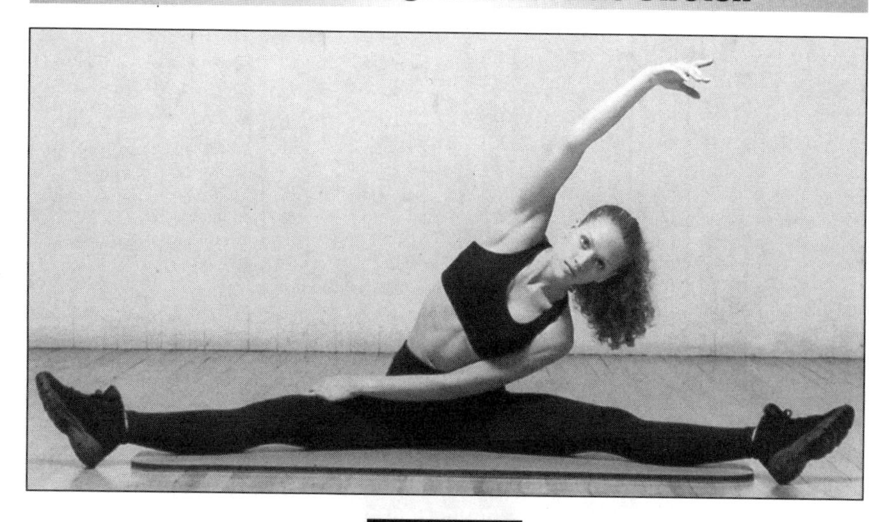

Static: Floor

While in the same spread position, instead of turning the upper body toward the foot, stay facing straight ahead. With your right arm, reach toward the ceiling and lean toward your left side and foot. Notice the position of the opposite arm and hand. Repeat on the opposite side.

Double Knee to the Shoulder

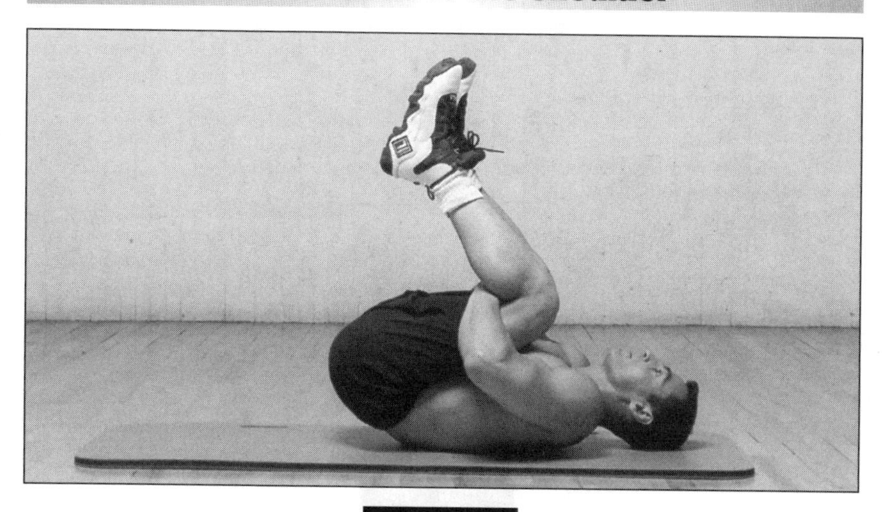

Static: Floor

Lie on your back and grab both legs behind the knees. Keep your back straight and pull both knees toward your shoulders. Maintain contact between the floor and your spine throughout the stretch.

Single Knee to the Shoulder

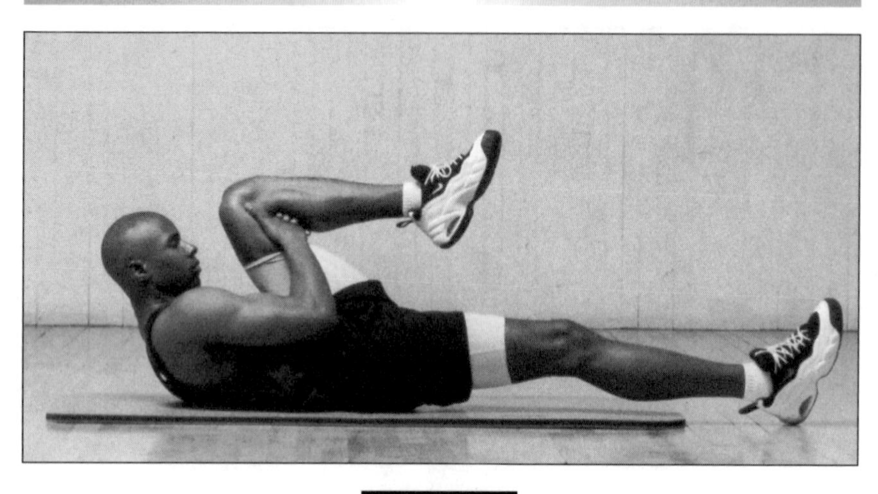

Static: Floor

Lie on your back and grab your left leg behind the knee. Slowly pull your left knee toward your left shoulder. To further stretch the back, lift your shoulders off the floor about four to six inches and hold the position.

Single Knee Progression—Bent Knee to Side

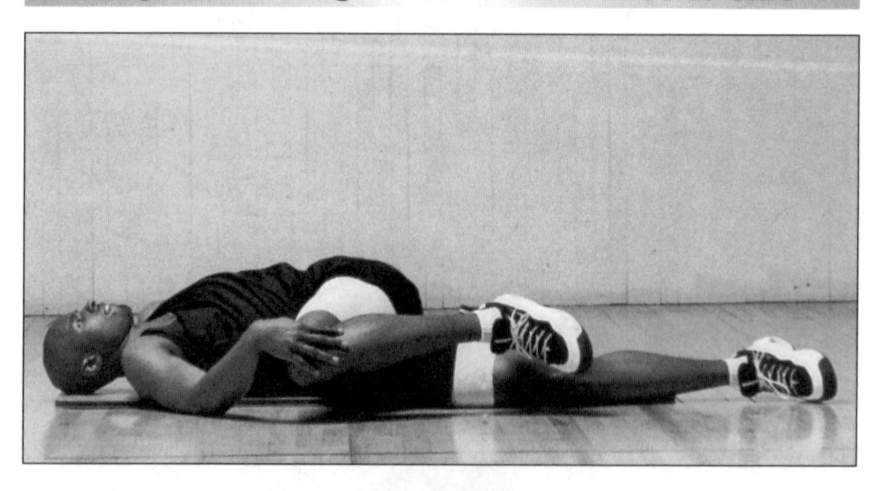

Static: Floor

For an excellent low back stretch, begin with the position described above, then return your shoulders to the floor, keeping the left knee bent and close to the shoulder. Take your right hand and gently pull the bent knee across your body to the right side. Make sure you keep both shoulders flat on the floor.

Single Knee Progression—Straight Leg to Side

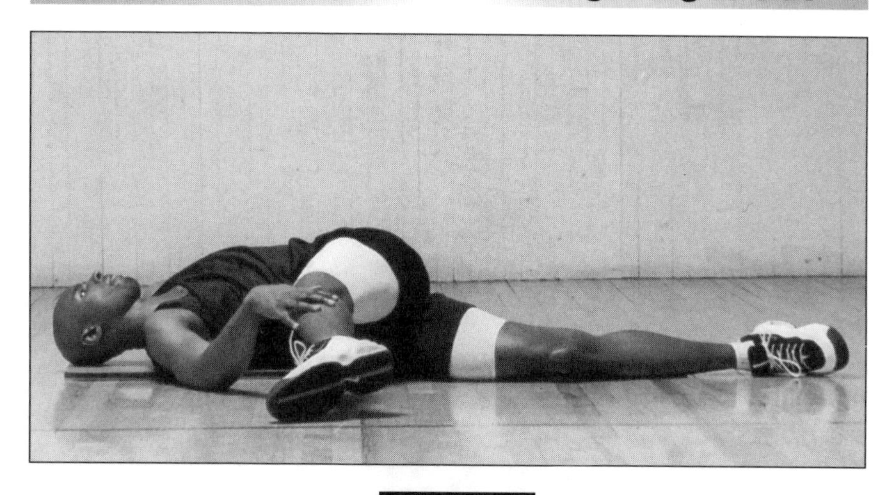

Static: Floor

With your knee back close to your shoulder, straighten your bent left leg and slowly lower it back down to the right side. Keep your shoulders flat on the floor.

Single Knee Progression—Crossed Leg Bent Knee

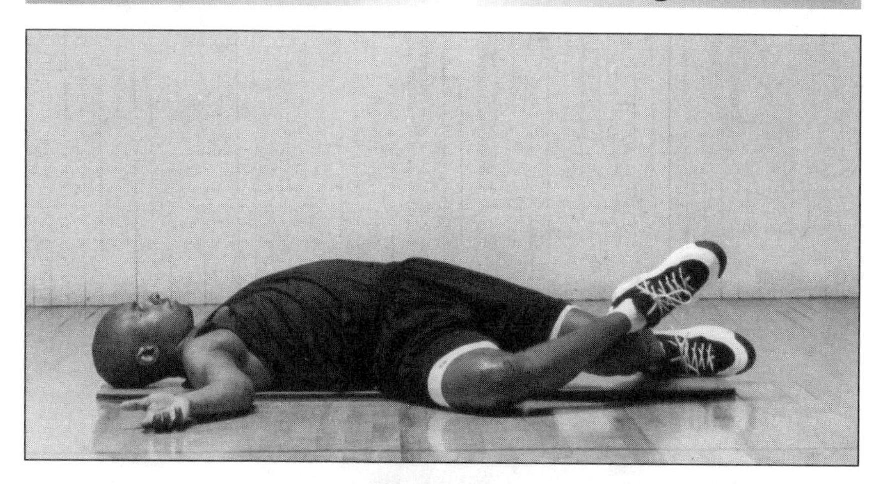

Static: Floor

Instead of pulling your bent knee to the side with your opposite hand, keep your left knee bent, but put your left foot flat on the floor. Cross your right leg over the left (right ankle positioned just above the left knee) and drop both legs to your right side. Again, keep both shoulders flat on the floor.

Inverted Hurdler

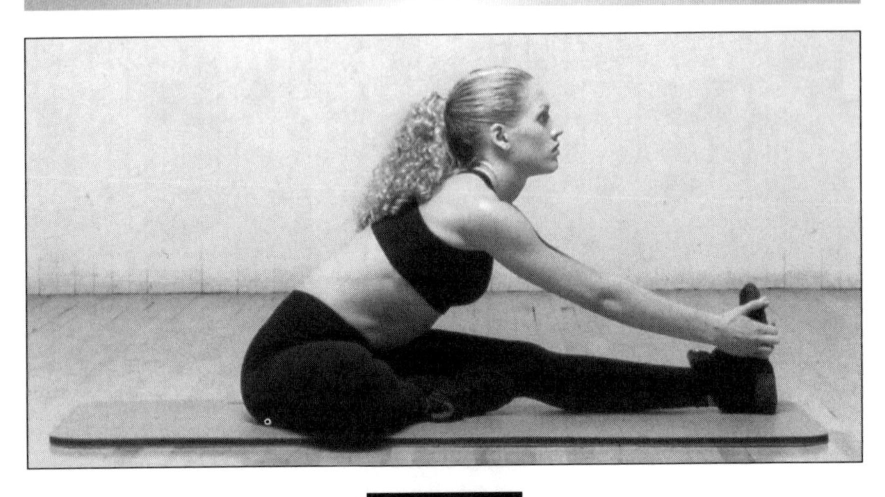

Static: Floor

Sitting on the floor, back straight and head up, extend your left leg. Place the sole of your right foot flat against the inside of your left leg. Focus your eyes on your left foot. Exhale and slowly lean out to your straight leg, keeping your head up.

Inverted Hurdler Progression: Reach "Over the Top"

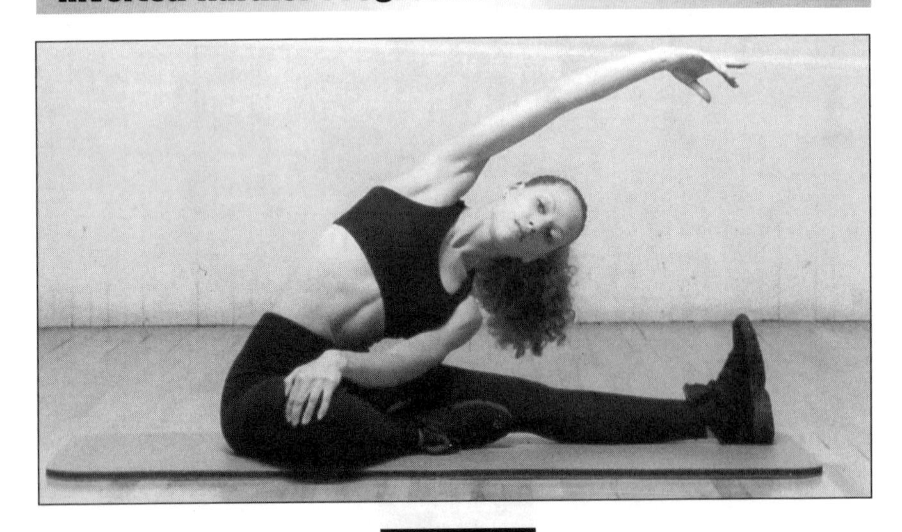

Static: Floor

Now place your left hand on your bent right knee. Look to the ceiling and reach "over the top" with your right hand toward the foot of your straight left leg. Notice the position of the shoulders.

Inverted Hurdler Progression: Pretzel

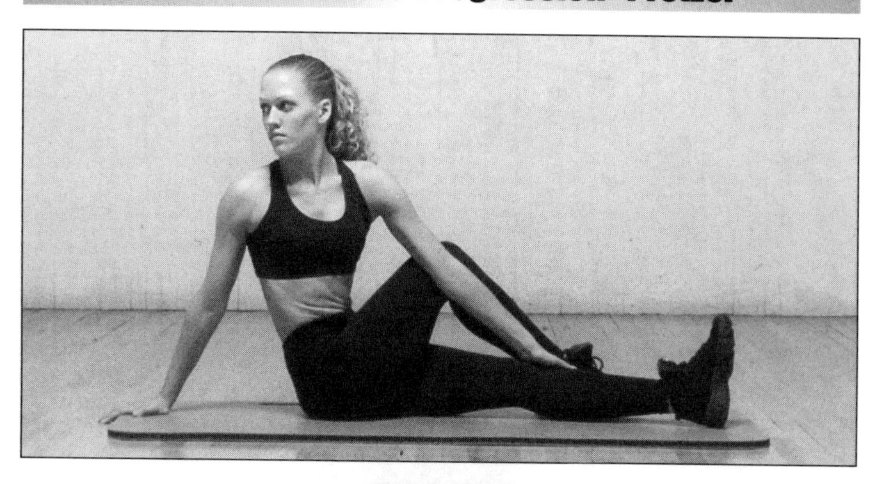

Static: Floor

While still in the inverted hurdler position, pick up your bent right leg and place it across your straight left leg, resting your right foot flat on the floor. Now place your left elbow on the outside of your right knee. Twist to the right. As your flexibility improves, reach around and "hook" your straight leg with your left hand (see above photo). This will give you greater leverage, enhancing the stretch.

Warning: The next three stretches are excellent abdominal stretches but carry a slight risk. Each of the stretches will require you to arch your back slightly. If hyperextending your back is uncomfortable for you or not recommended by your doctor, skip these three stretches and choose those more appropriate for you.

Abdominal Stretch

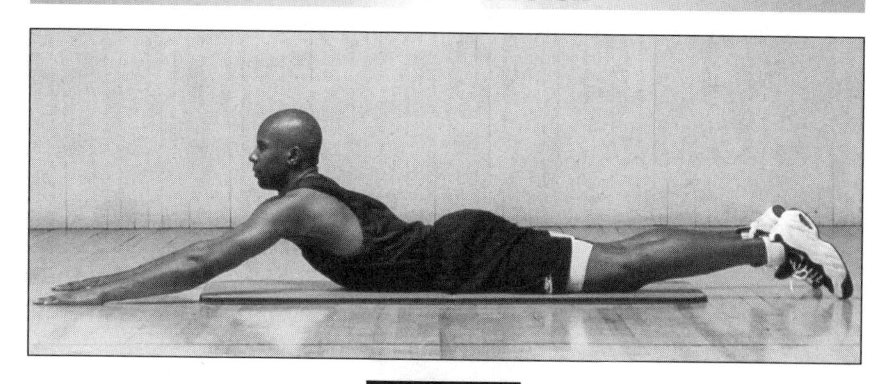

Static: Floor

Lying on your stomach, extend your arms overhead, hands on the floor. Gently lift your upper body off the floor.

Abdominal Stretch Progression: Elbows Under

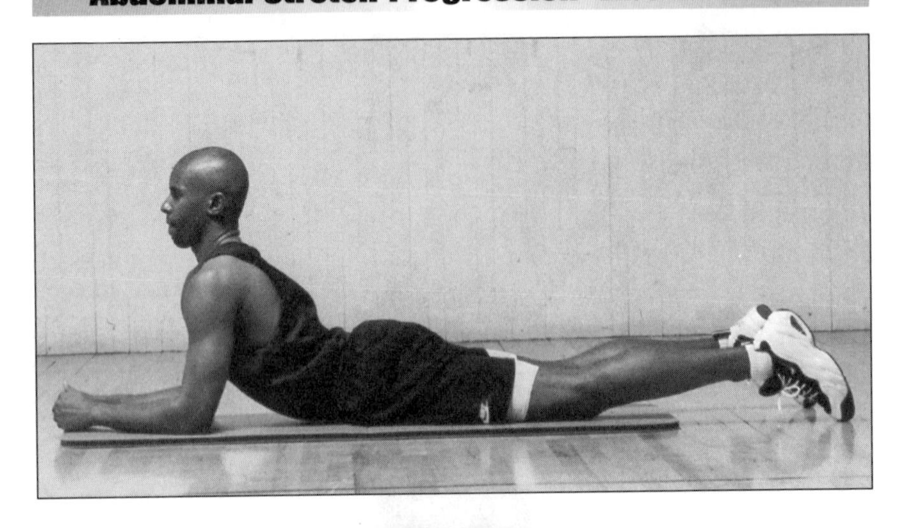

Static: Floor

While lying on your stomach, lift your upper body and hold the position, supporting yourself with your elbows.

Prone Twist

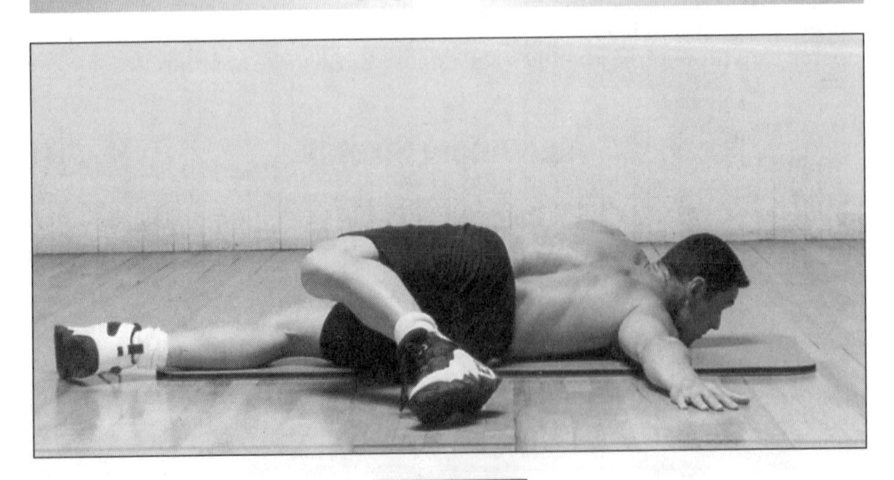

Static: Floor

Still lying on your stomach, extend your arms perpendicular to your body. Lift your left leg and twist as if attempting to touch your right hand with your left foot. Keep both shoulders on the floor.

Dynamic Stretching Guidelines

- These stretches involve dynamic, and sometimes rapid, stretching of the muscles. Compared to the ballistic nature of most sports movements, however, these stretches pose minimal risk. If an athlete can't handle the rigors of a dynamic stretch, she is most certainly at risk during intense competition. In contrast, the general fitness enthusiast should approach these stretches with caution or avoid them entirely.

Trunk and Low Torso Stretches

Punter's Stretch

Dynamic: Standing

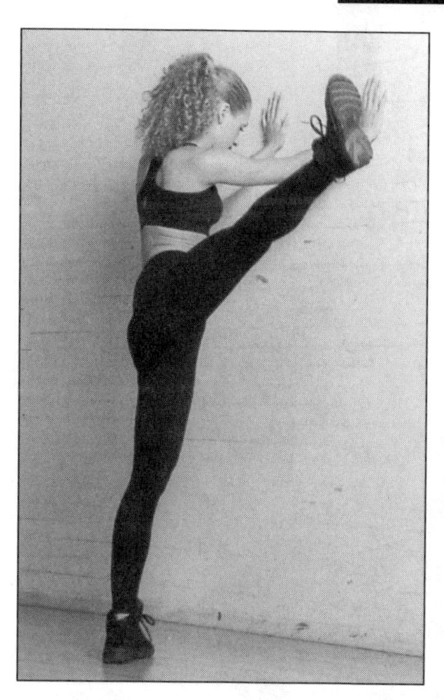

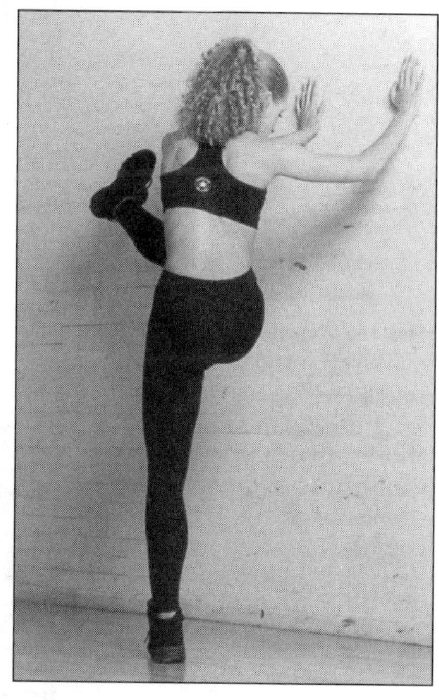

Standing on your left leg with your left foot pointing toward a wall, place both hands on the wall, keeping your shoulders facing the wall. Slowly lift your right leg to the side (laterally). After a brief hesitation and in one motion, pivot your left foot and hips and "drive" your right leg through as if punting a football. You should feel a stretch in your low back and buttocks.

Full Range Trunk Twist

Dynamic: Standing

Place your feet slightly wider than shoulder-width apart with your hands on your hips. Slowly rotate your upper body clockwise, being careful to avoid extreme hyperextension (arching) of the low back. Continue for 5 to 10 revolutions, then repeat in the other direction.

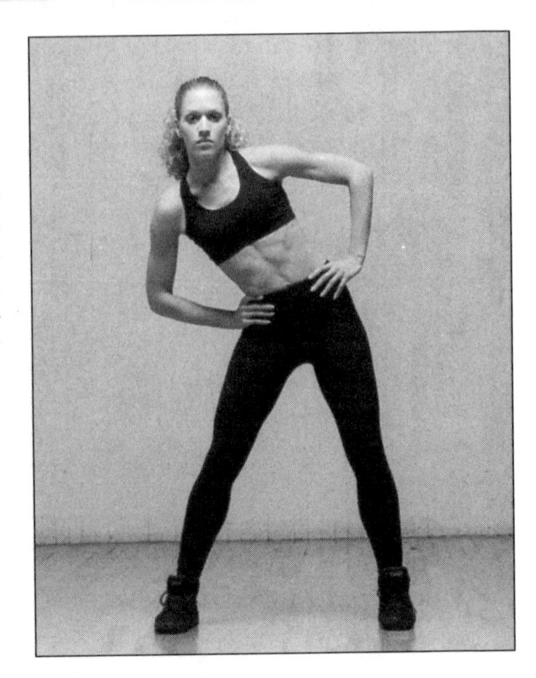

Short Range Trunk Twist

Dynamic: Standing

The only difference between this stretch and the Full Range Trunk Twist is that the feet are together and the movement is abbreviated and rapid. With your hands on your hips, you should have the feeling that you are "pushing" your hips around in a circle.

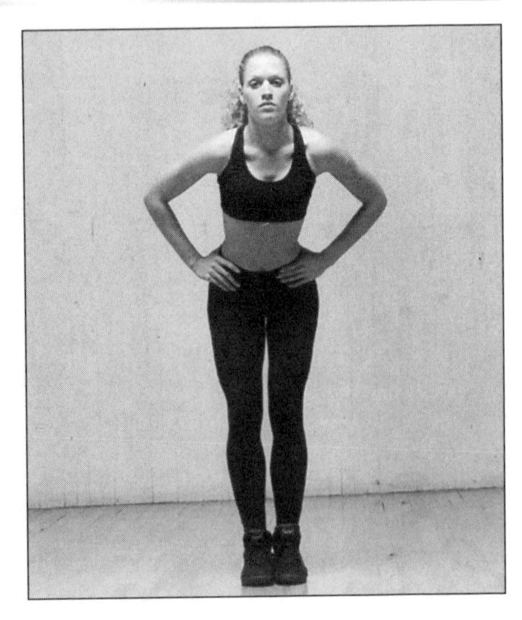

Hanging Twist

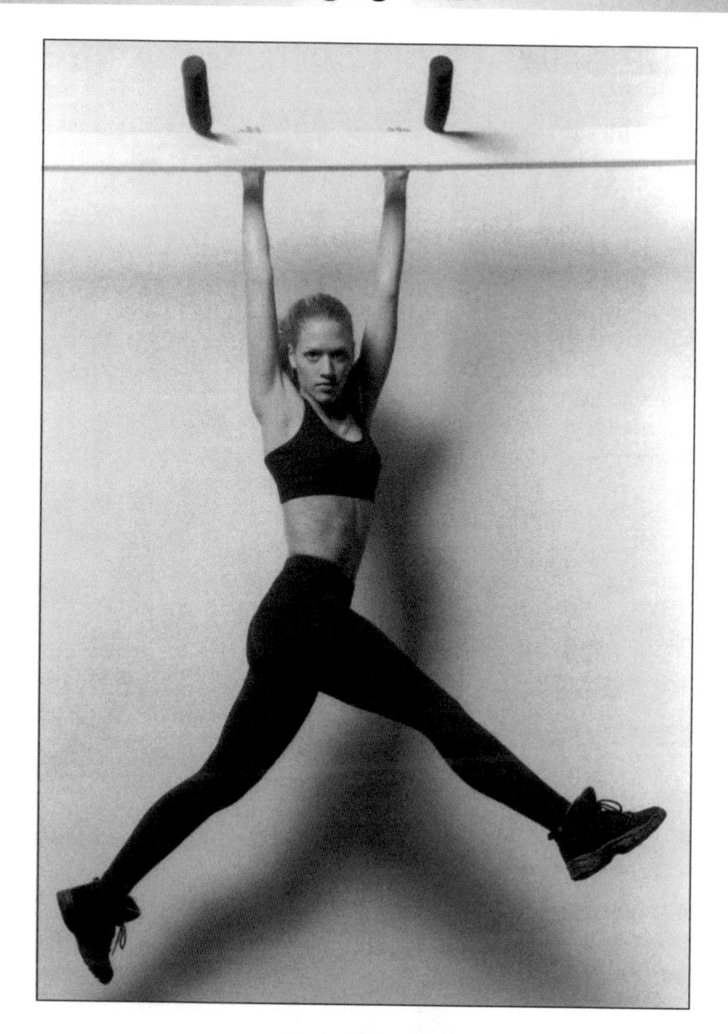

Dynamic: Standing

For this exercise, you'll need a chin-up bar high enough to allow for full extension of your body without your feet touching the floor. Take a comfortable grip, hands approximately shoulder-width apart, and slowly start rotating your trunk from side to side, using your legs for momentum.

Side Bend With Broomstick

Dynamic: Standing

Place your feet in a comfortable but considerably wider than shoulder-width stance. Hold a broomstick across your shoulders, taking a wide grip. From this position, the exercise can be done as either a dynamic or static stretch. The dynamic stretch involves continuous movement from side to side, while the static stretch requires a pause of 10 seconds minimum on each side.

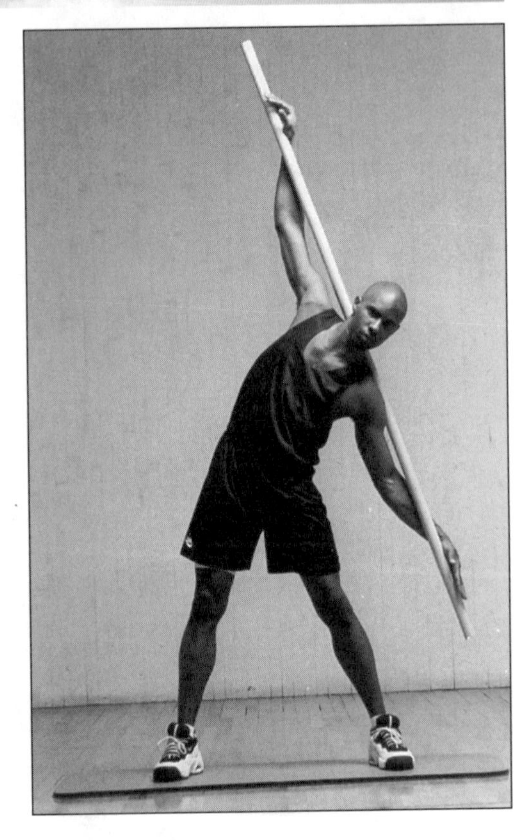

Trunk Rotation With Broomstick

Dynamic: Standing

Place the broomstick across your shoulders and your feet shoulder-width apart. Rotate your upper body to the left and right several times. You can also perform this exercise while seated.

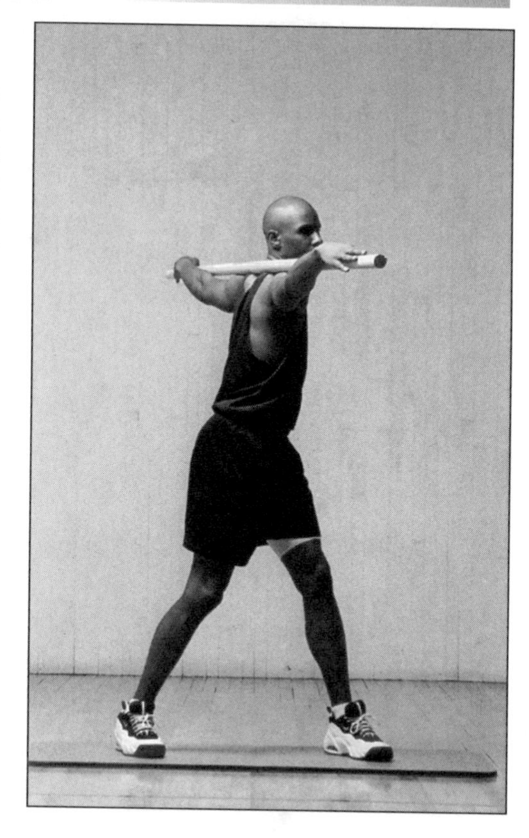

Tennis Serve Stretch With Broomstick

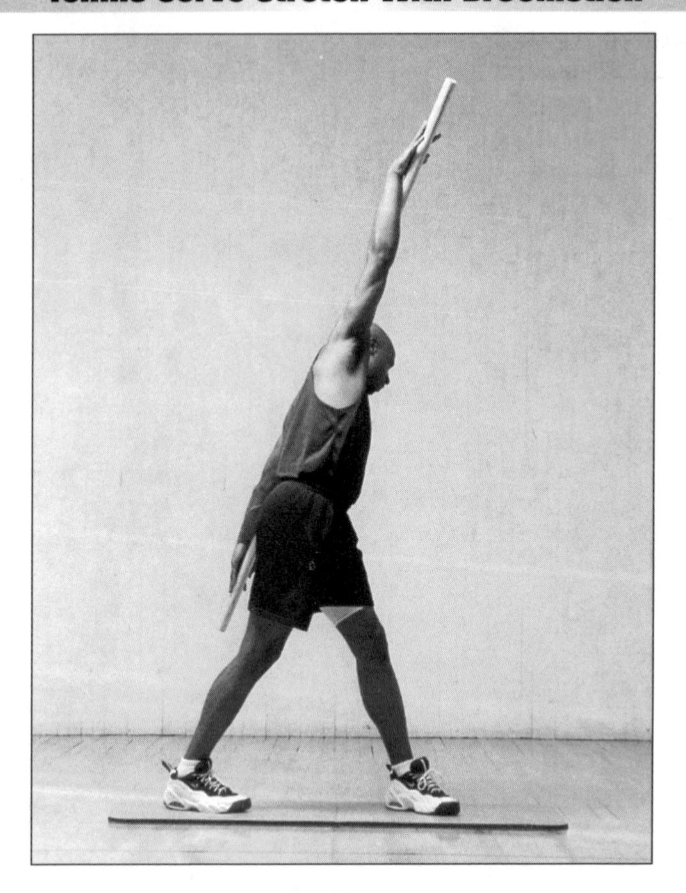

Dynamic: Standing

Keeping the broomstick across your shoulders and your arms extended, place your feet wider than shoulder-width apart. Bending your knees slightly, twist slowly and point your left hand at your right heel. Moving slowly and continuously, repeat to the opposite side.

4

Training Guidelines

Defying skeptics, the fitness trend in America continues to grow. An increasing number of people are interested in improving their health. Unfortunately, fad programs promising to "whip the participant into shape" through strenuous exercise and trendy diets can lead to new problems. Fortunately, you can reduce many physical complications by simply exercising regularly and safely.

Training can both build up and break down systems in the body; you must understand both processes to create the most effective program possible. Improper training can lead to injury; intelligent training emphasizes the prevention of injuries. For example, close to half of all runners will at some point develop knee and back problems. Many factors can lead to muscular imbalances: improper mechanics, inadequate strength, inadequate flexibility, inappropriate equipment such as the wrong shoes, deficient training techniques, or overtraining. These imbalances make you more vulnerable to injury. Eliminating or avoiding imbalances begins at the core. So before you get started on developing your center of power, note a few precautions.

This manual contains many abdominal and low back exercises. We have identified those exercises which may be "chancy" for novice fitness enthusiasts, but we cannot account for all the different body types, specific diseases, injuries, and mechanical deviations that exist. Therefore, if you have concerns with this—or any other new program—consult your physician, coach, trainer, or a qualified fitness instructor both to determine if any of the drills you choose pose a risk to you and at which level you should begin.

Once you ascertain your appropriate starting level, you must follow a proper training progression, maintain correct technique, and establish a frequent routine to gain the most benefits from the time and effort you invest. First, learn and master the steps of each exercise before attempting heavier resistance or increasing the volume.

Never sacrifice technique for added resistance or repetitions! If you deviate from correct technique, you may rehearse bad movement patterns, develop muscle imbalances (asymmetrical strength development), or incur an injury. The only way to maximize your workout is to adhere strictly to the drill descriptions.

Second, begin with light resistance and low repetition training, then gradually build up to a greater resistance and/or higher repetition routine. This manual models safe progressions, but *you* must judge whether or not your technique allows for advancement.

Third, exercise often enough to create a significant effect. Initially, we recommend that you exercise four or five days per week for several months. Once you have achieved your goal—"washboard abs," elimination of low back pain, improved athletic control, greater strength and power, or the like—you can decrease the duration (number of repetitions per set) and the frequency of your training to as little as twice a week and still maintain your accomplishments. (*Note*: The New York Knicks currently employ a "three on, one off" routine, training the center of power for three days straight then taking a one-day rest.)

Frequency refers to *how often* you train the center of power, while duration refers to the *length* of a workout (measured by the number of sets and repetitions per session). Intensity is the *level of difficulty*, which is determined by adding or subtracting resistance or varying the speed of the exercise.

After achieving your goals, you can get away with fewer workouts but not with lower intensity. If you decrease the intensity you will experience a rapid *detraining* effect. Months of hard work and dramatic accomplishments can be quickly lost once you stop training. Likewise, sporadic exercise will not fully develop your center of power in the first place, nor will it enhance performance or decrease the incidence or severity of low back pain. Only those who make the commitment to a lifestyle of regular training will reap its benefits.

Unless otherwise stated, observe the following precautions. Remember, this book cannot account for varying levels of fitness among its readers, and there will always be exceptions to the rule. Although we may strongly recommend an exercise for an athlete's training program, it may be ill-advised for the general population.

- In general, avoid bilateral (double) straight leg lifts, straight-leg sit-ups, Roman Chair exercises, or any exercise that arches the low back. The psoas muscles run from the upper legs, through the pelvis, and attach to the low back. When the legs are in a straight position, the psoas muscles are placed in high tension and pull on the low back. If you are free from back pain, try a little experiment. Lie on the

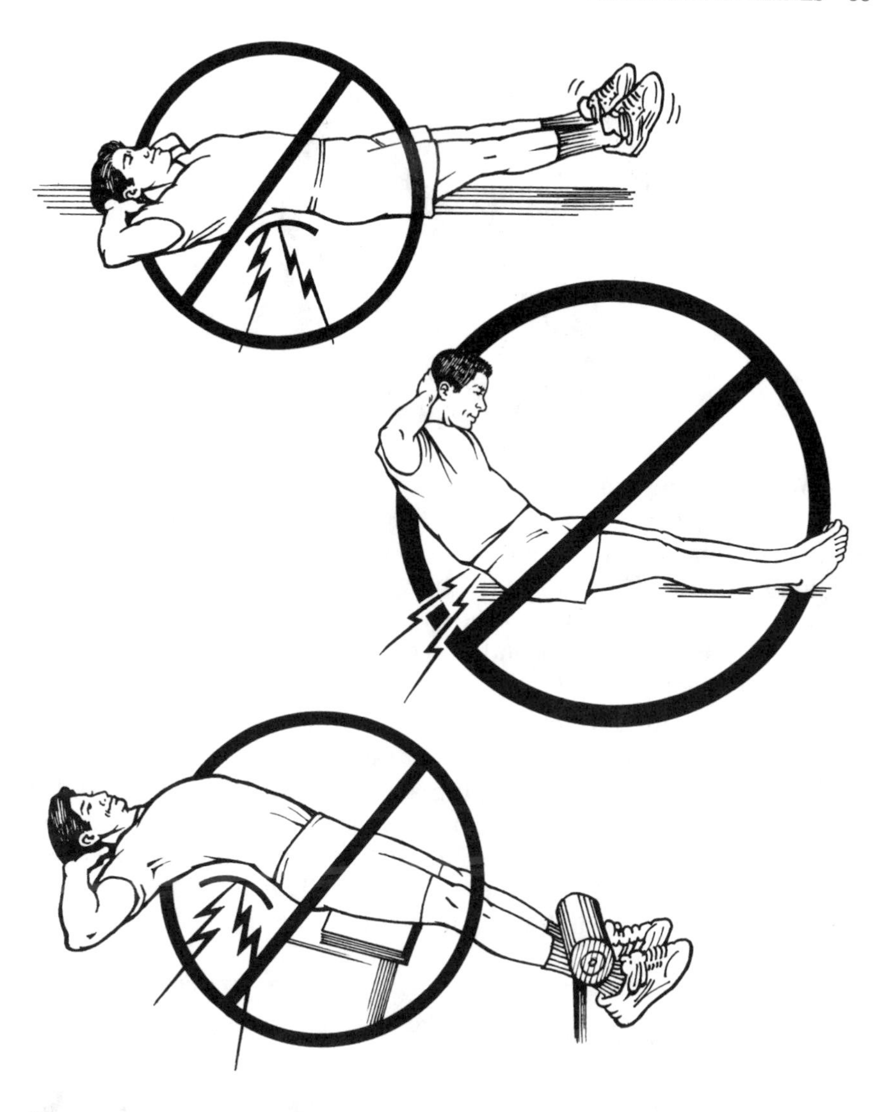

floor on your back with your legs extended. Slowly raise your legs off the floor a couple of inches and try to slide your hand under your low back. If there is a space between the floor and your low back, then your spine is in hyperextension and therefore subjected to potentially dangerous stress. Avoid exercises that place your spine in severe hyperextension like this.

• Extreme flexion of the spine, the opposite of back hyperextension, also requires caution. This is one of the drawbacks of any "full" sit-up exercise. The abdominal muscles work primarily within a 0- to 45-degree range of motion; any movement beyond 45 degrees forces the strong hip flexor and psoas muscles to assume much of the work.

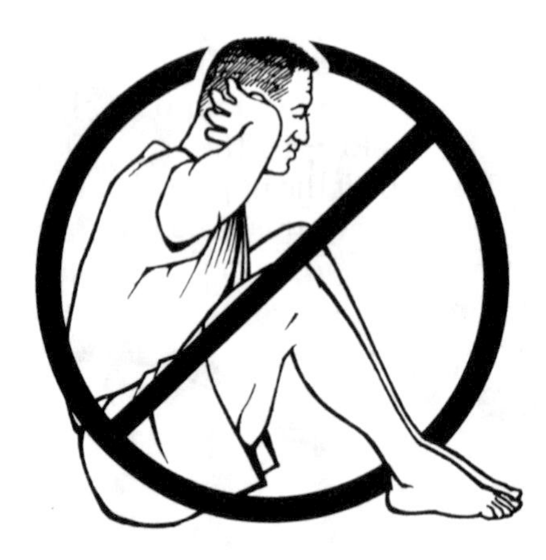

If you are curling completely forward, we say that your spine is in "full flexion." If the spine is in full flexion then *intra-discal* pressure increases, which can cause problems in individuals with degenerating lumbar discs. Unless you're involved in sprinting, jumping, kicking, or any other activity that requires ballistic and explosive flexing of the hips, isolate your abs and concentrate on those exercises within the 0- to 45-degree range.

• Because of their weight, or resistance, the position of your hands and arms makes a significant difference in how much stress you place on the working muscles and, ultimately, in the effectiveness of the exercise. The farther the resistance is located from the point of axis, the greater the demand on the abdominals. The point of axis varies, depending on the exercise, but it is generally located between the hip and the waist. The following photos show an athlete performing a

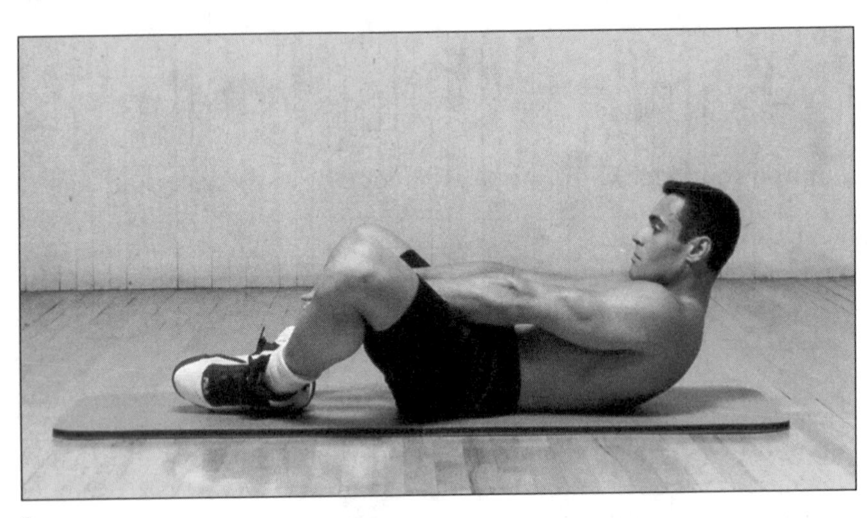

a

curl-up, using three different arm positions. The axis point for a curl-up is located at the waist. In photo *a* on page 54, the arms are forward, and their weight is close to the axis. In this position, the abdominals work less hard to lift the upper body. Photo *b* below shows a mid-range arm position, moving the resistance farther from the axis, thereby placing a greater demand on the abdominals to lift the upper body. Finally, in photo *c*, with the arms behind the head, the resistance is even farther from the axis point located at the waist, placing the greatest amount of stress on the abs.

If you are new to abdominal training or your abs more closely resemble a Jell-O cube than a washboard, you should start all your

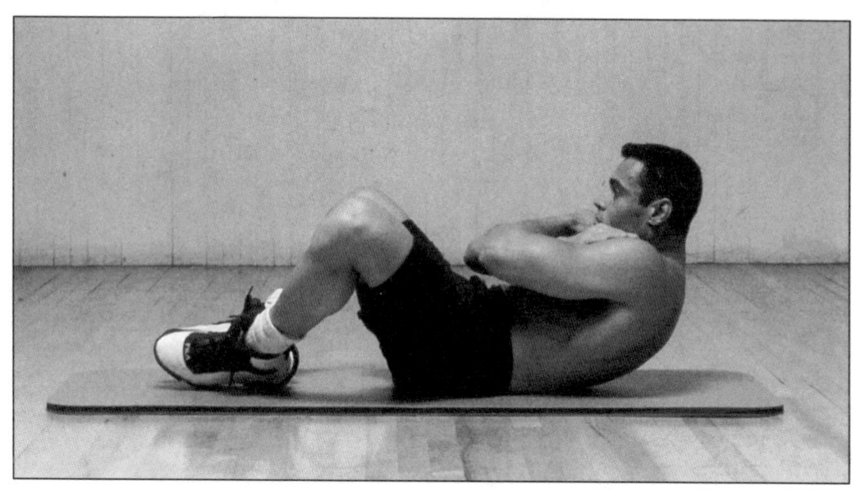

b

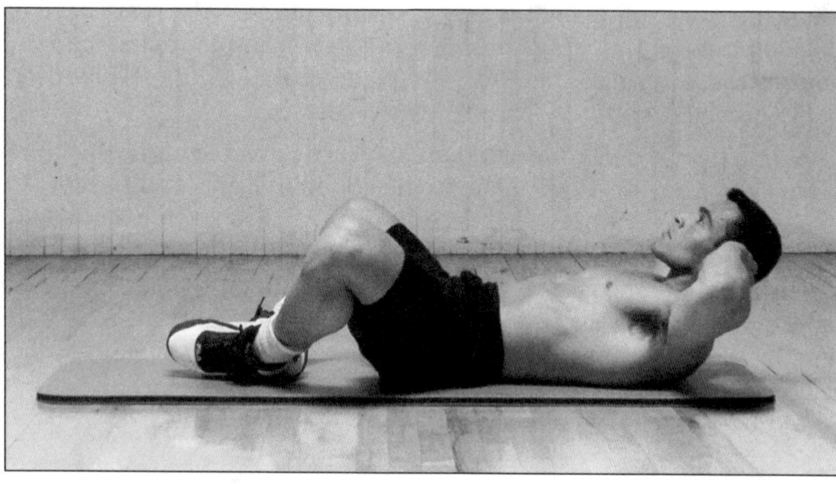

c

exercises with your arms close to the axis point. As your strength develops, progressively move the arms to more demanding positions. Never, however, compromise technique when determining the correct position for your arms! This is especially important as fatigue sets in. The photo below shows the exerciser pulling on his head and neck in an effort to squeeze out a few additional reps. Unfortunately, he is at risk of injury, especially as fatigue begins to interfere with correct technique. Rather than risk a neck injury, he should simply reposition his arms from the more demanding locations to a position closer to the axis point.

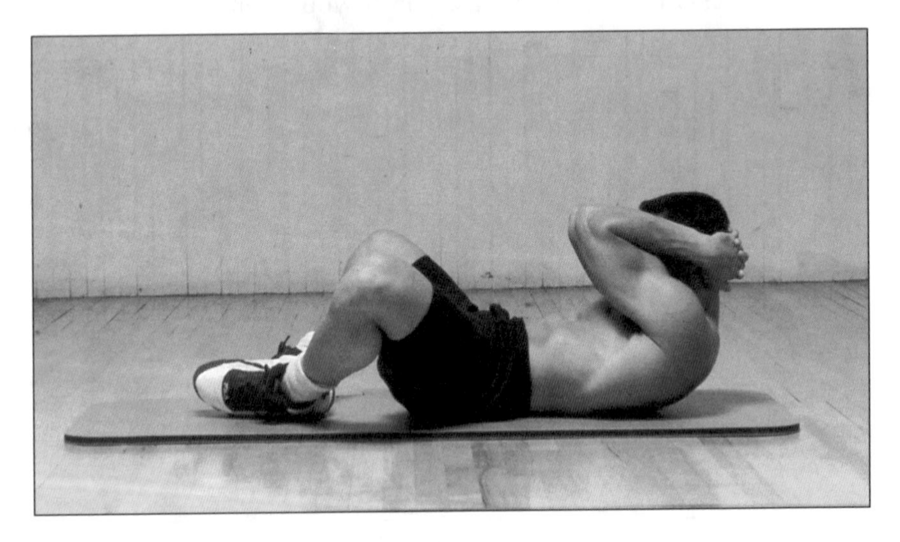

• As your strength develops and you start to transform that Jell-O cube into rock, you might feel the need to increase the resistance by placing a weight, such as a phone book or iron plate, first on your chest, then eventually behind your head. Again, do *not* sacrifice technique in an attempt to increase resistance.

• The position of your legs also plays a major role in the effectiveness of an exercise. Refer again to the abdominal axis point examples (see pages 54-55), only this time, let's discuss the function of the legs. The farther the weight of your legs from the point of axis, the greater *leverage* you can generate to lift your upper body. Therefore, if you are just beginning an abdominal program, you may want to experiment with different leg positions as dictated by your present level of abdominal strength. (See photos on page 57.)

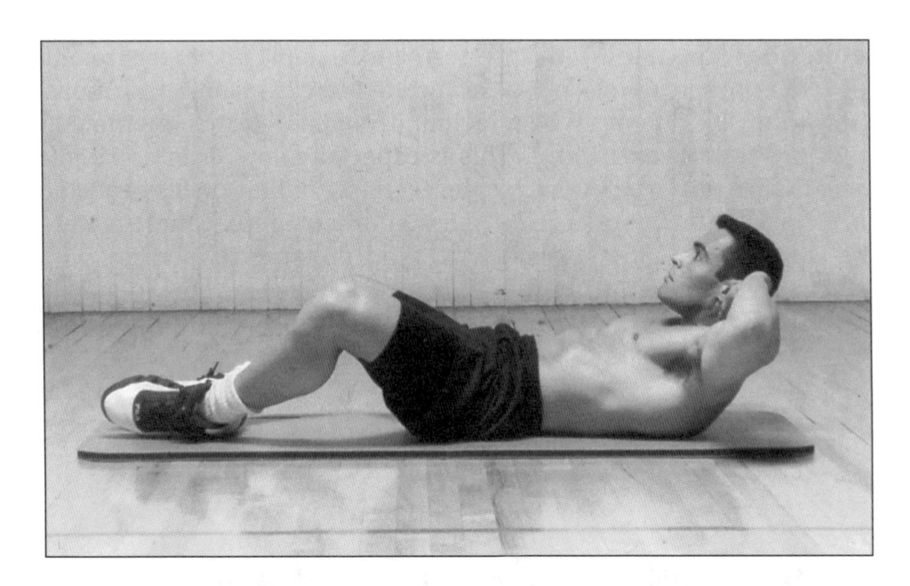

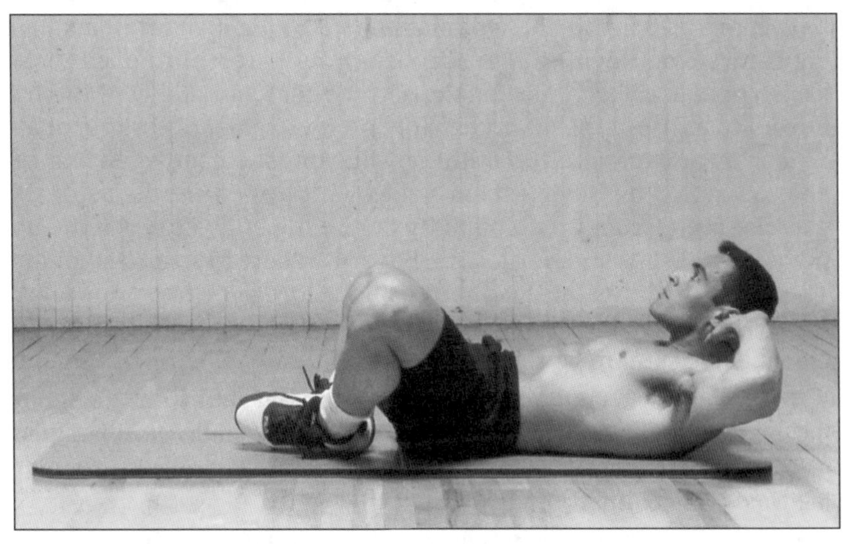

• Many fitness enthusiasts just starting out may not have the abdominal strength to perform an unassisted exercise and therefore are quickly discouraged from continuing a program. If positioning the arms close to the point of axis and extending the legs doesn't give enough assistance to the abdominals, try these options. First, try holding a light weight in your hands to provide additional weight closer to the axis (see photo on page 58).

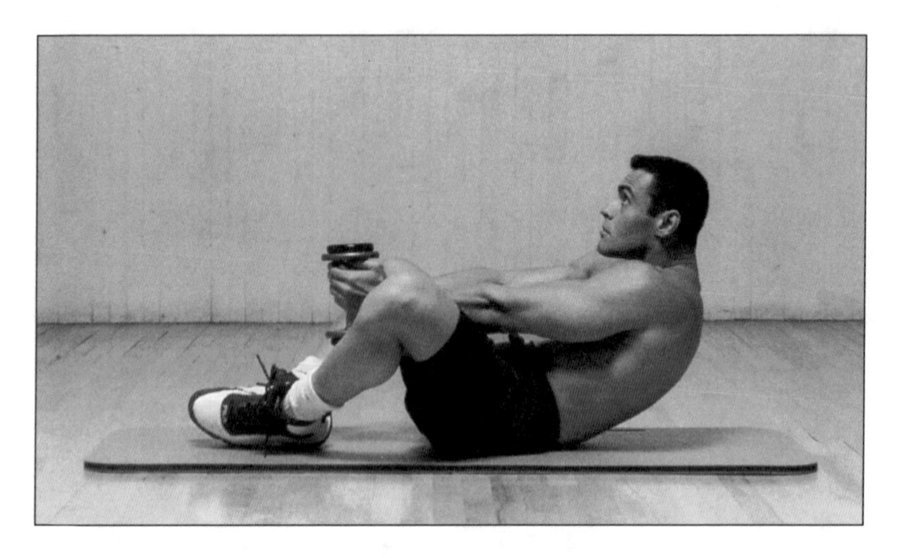

If you are still having difficulty, hold onto a partner's hands and have him assist in the lift. Avoid pulling with your own arms; instead, concentrate on isolating your abs while your partner provides gentle assistance. If all else fails, anchoring the feet and allowing the hip flexors to assist in the lift is certainly preferable to no workout at all. When you anchor your feet, either by hooking them under an immovable object or by having them held by a partner, the focus of the exercise shifts from predominantly on the upper abs to both the upper and lower abs and hip flexors. But still adhere to strict technique. The range of motion at the hip remains below 45 degrees, the lower back is supported, not arched, and you can concentrate on the specific muscles you're working.

- If your goal is general fitness, that is, to develop strength and to flatten your abs, perform the exercises in a slow and controlled manner. "Jerking" allows you to take advantage of momentum, decreasing the work required of your abs.

- Remember, we recommend the drills outlined in chapter 8 primarily for the experienced athlete. The general fitness enthusiast should not attempt these more demanding exercises.

- During all exercises, keep your breathing rhythmic and natural. Never hold your breath. Typically, you should exhale during the contraction, or lifting phase, and inhale during the relaxation, or lowering, phase. We recommend that, if at all possible, you perform the exercises in front of a mirror. This will provide you with immediate visual feedback, helping you to more quickly develop proper technique.

Training Guidelines

To ensure maximum center of power development, follow these guidelines.

- Always fatigue the weaker regions first. Train your abdominals in the following order:
  1. Obliques
  2. Lower abs
  3. Upper abs
- Because the upper abdominals assist with movements in the lower and oblique abdominal region, it is important *not* to fatigue the upper abs first. This would decrease the productivity of the other muscles of the core. In order to achieve synergism, or complete development, of the center of power, do not limit yourself to working just the strong muscles; rather, incorporate all muscles of the region into your routine.
- Keep workouts balanced. Always train opposing muscle groups equally to prevent muscle imbalances. For example, the low back muscles are opposite to the abdominals.
- Maintain a tight contraction throughout the entire set. Keep rest to a minimum between sets, and never rest between exercises *during* a set.
- If you are just beginning an abdominal program, experiment with different arm and leg positions until you have the strength to perform the correct movement unassisted.
- As a general rule, limit the range of motion of the abdominals to 45 degrees or less. Exceptions: some of the more advanced exercises that use the psoas and other secondary muscles to facilitate the movement (see chapter 8).
- Because the abdominals can be easily fatigued, it's easy to succumb to poor technique in order to "crunch out" a few extra repetitions. *Never* sacrifice technique!
- Choose a variety of exercises and mix them up periodically. Attacking the trunk and low torso from different angles will ensure total development, allow for recovery of opposing muscles, and stave off boredom.

- Always include a comprehensive warm-up and cooldown routine in any training program.
- To keep your program progressive, as your strength increases gradually increase both the number of repetitions per set and the number of sets per session. Approach adding an external resistance (e.g., telephone books, iron plates, wrist weights, and the like) with extreme caution. As always, *never* sacrifice form for added sets, repetitions, or resistance!
- The cadence, or speed, of the movement will vary, depending on the ballistic nature of the exercise and the range of motion involved. As a general rule, do most strength and toning exercises slowly and the power exercises at greater speed. Look for the suggested cadence under the exercise name. You may want to try varying the speed throughout the movement. For example, two seconds up, pause for one second, then four seconds down.

Slow Slow cadence, one repetition per one or more seconds.

Moderate Medium cadence, one to two repetitions per second.

Fast Fast cadence, greater than two repetitions per second.

Explosive Explosive cadence, the number of repetitions per second will vary, depending upon the range of motion of the exercise. Used mainly with medicine ball exercises.

- Remember, your gains will be quickly lost if you stop training.

5

Trunk Stabilization and Balance Exercises

Have you ever ambled around a health club and noticed some large and colorful balls lying about and wondered how the nursery's toys made their way into the weight room? I must admit that on more than one occasion I caught myself dribbling, passing, and smacking my fellow exercise enthusiasts in the head with youthful merriment only to be scolded by the resident physical therapist and sternly instructed to leave the "TheraBalls" alone. While these balls have many uses, their original intent, and our primary concern, is the many trunk stabilization, flexibility, and strengthening exercises that you can perform safely and effectively with such a simple apparatus. But before we start bouncing on balls, let's examine the value of a stabilized core.

THE VALUE OF A STABILIZED CORE

The abdominal and low back muscles play a dominant role in controlling posture, lumbar (lower spine) stabilization, and total body balance. Consequently, a well-developed core will decrease the likelihood and severity of injury and encourage more efficient movement. Lifting, good posture, balance, walking, swinging a golf club, running, and dunking a basketball would be impossible without the effective involvement of the core muscles.

Unfortunately, today's sedentary lifestyle has intensified the breakdown of this very important structural system in the body. Our society, which we think of as fast-paced, is in fact physically immobile. In years past, fatigue was the result of a hard day's work in the field or the factory. The physical-labor-related fatigue of our grandparents has been replaced by stress-related fatigue. Nowadays, emotional stress prevails and is often the result of spending endless hours in traffic jams, retyping 20-page proposals lost to killer computer viruses, or agonizing over which designer coffee to sip or which one of several thousand television programs to watch.

Movement is essential to life, yet we are living in a motionless society. Too many of us roll out of bed in the morning, slam down a bagel and a cup of "joe," commute to work, sit, commute home, sit in front of the tube, return to bed, then repeat. It's no wonder that our core becomes weak, tense, and less effective. Prolonged inactivity, poor physical conditioning, extended periods of sitting or standing in awkward positions, and years of poor posture eventually lead to structural deterioration. Smaller weaker muscles must compensate for the decline of their larger partners, resulting in muscle imbalances, tight joints, low back and other joint injuries, and, ultimately, a total system degeneration.

Visiting the doctor has become the accepted mode of dealing with physical problems in our quick-fix mentality. This passive approach alienates us from our own health and fitness potential. Exercise, in contrast, will help to maintain proper and efficient functioning of all systems in the body. Freedom of movement in harmony with the body's design, without the constraints of poor posture, will help eliminate inferior function, thereby enhancing health and well-being. We must regain control of our own fitness and performance potential. If we take control of balance, stability, and posture, motion will become efficient, leading to controlled performance with a minimum of wasted energy. This conservation of energy enables us to deal better with physical and emotional stress and enables the athlete to perform at a high intensity for a longer duration with less fatigue.

Far Eastern philosophers have been preaching these concepts for thousands of years. Trunk and torso stabilization techniques are as much a daily ritual for them as are eating and sleeping. There are many philosophically based techniques that share a similar view. That is, enhance the quality of life through maximizing efficiency of physical function. Eastern martial artists routinely concentrate the greatest percentage of their training time on the development of the "Hara" (the core), the physical center of our being.

Relaxation of the muscles made possible by a strong core allows for greater freedom of movement, more power in movement, fewer extraneous movements, and, most importantly, conservation of energy through efficient movement. Only after achieving this ability to channel energy can you begin to realize your tremendous physical potential.

Controlled body movement is also a prerequisite of accuracy of skill. Indeed, accuracy begins at the core. Moreover, the power devel-

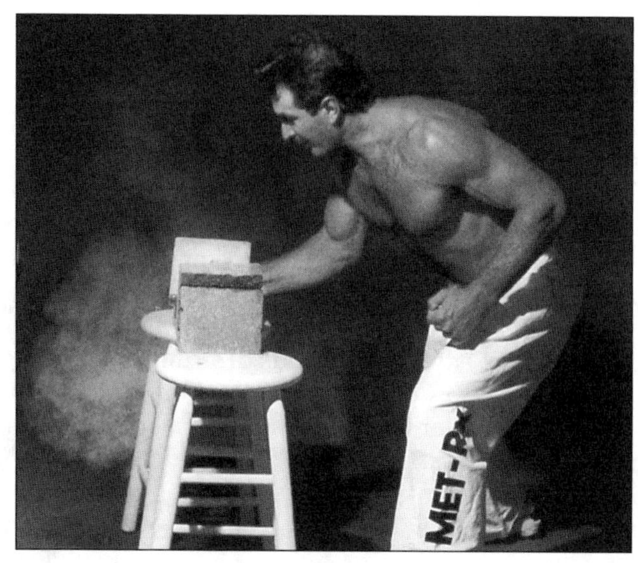

© Ron Barker

oped in the core must eventually be able to travel through the musculoskeletal system to the more precision-oriented extremities (distal musculature).

TRANSFER OF POWER

Your training goal is to transport the tremendous power potential of the core toward the extremities through progressively smaller and weaker muscles without a loss of energy. For example, if you were to lock your elbow and wrist and extend your index finger, then attempt to push your friend, the force generated from the pelvic muscles will efficiently transfer from your core through your straight arm to your fingertip with little energy loss. The resulting push would at least cause some discomfort—if not knock your friend off-balance (see figure *a* on page 64). If, however, you were to bend one of the joints along the chain such as your elbow, the force generated by the core would dissipate through the bend in the elbow. In other words, the strong muscles of the core become less effective and the resulting push might resemble nothing more than an aggressive tickle (see figure *b* on page 64).

Remember the example of the sprinter whose shoulder, hip, knee, and ankle are in alignment? (See page 6.) In this position during the push phase of the stride, the sprinter can more efficiently channel the force generated by lower body muscles through the center of power to the upper body, and vice versa. It takes a strong core to achieve this alignment.

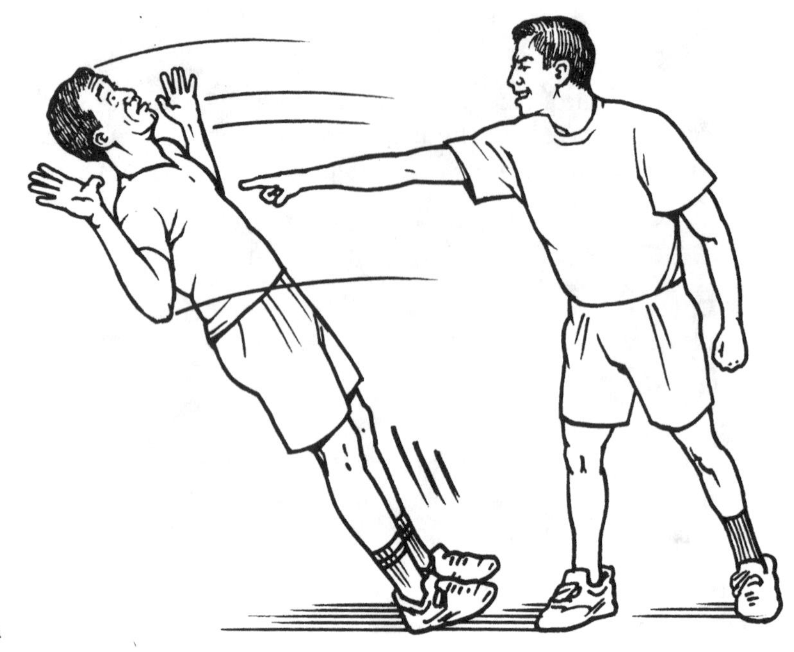

a

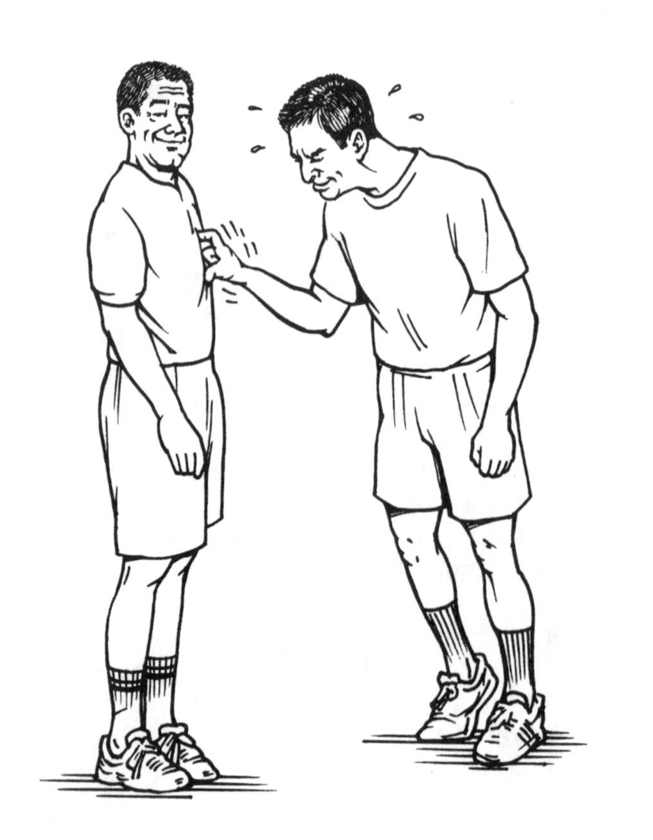

b

BALANCE

Balance is the result of correct body alignment. The proper relationship between the core and the legs, arms, feet, hands, and head is essential to achieving correct body alignment.

Characteristics of Good Balance

From an athletic perspective, someone who is balanced typically demonstrates the following traits:

1. The knees are flexed, rather than straight, creating a low center of gravity.
2. The base of support is wide with the feet usually parallel.
3. Body weight is on the balls of the feet.
4. The center of gravity is dynamic. That is, the athlete continually uses rapid, yet controlled, motion to respond to sudden changes of direction.

The ability to accurately adjust to changes in your position or to unstable equilibrium and to understand your limitations in the constant battle with gravity indicates accomplished balance—a trait most great athletes possess.

Dynamic Balance

Maintaining balance and stability is a dynamic process. Without any conscious effort, your body's muscular system is continually contracting and relaxing in order to sustain a sitting, standing, walking, running, or any other imaginable posture. Your body is continually trying to attain a state of equilibrium. Several mechanisms within your body work to achieve this aim. Two of the more pertinent sources of feedback include

1. the *vestibular apparatus* within the inner ear, which relays information to the central nervous system concerning the body's spatial awareness, including any deviations from the vertical position; and

2. *proprioceptors* within the muscles and joints such as the *muscle spindle* and *golgi tendon organ,* which sense the magnitude and speed of a stretched muscle and changes in joint angles. These sensors provide input necessary to make immediate and essential adjustments in balance.

A good example of your receptors at work is that disturbing feeling of just beginning to nod off only to be abruptly jerked back to reality. Imagine sitting in front of a roaring fire in your big easy chair. While perusing Dostoyevsky's *Crime and Punishment*, your eyes begin to close and your head slowly drops forward. The muscle spindles in the back of your neck sense this stretch placed on the neck muscles and quickly make a correction by firing those muscles and returning your head to an upright position—a rude reminder that your receptor mechanisms are hard at work. From a stabilization, balance, and postural standpoint, refining your proprioceptor sensors will enhance fitness and athletic performance as well as decrease the chance of injury.

POSTURE

For years, our parents implored us to "stand straight" and "sit tall." What's so important about posture, anyway?

The Importance of Good Posture

Poor posture can affect balance profoundly. Keep in mind that you can transfer force most effectively through a straight line. Obviously, there are natural curvatures throughout the body but generally you should strive for straight lines between *segments* particularly during the push or explosive phase of a movement. A person with poor posture is lacking that straight line. The preferred path of force transfer is through the skeletal system. Poor posture, however, causes detours in the force transfer because the smaller and weaker muscles outside the core must act as the force conduit. Much wasted energy results, and subsequent, and usually more severe, breakdowns are inescapable. This can lead to countless mechanical and structural problems.

Postural Problems

Poor posture over many years will most certainly result in problems ranging from slight discomfort to pain so severe that surgery becomes the only relief. The following figures highlight two of the most common abnormalities associated with poor posture.

Anterior Pelvic Tilt

The figure below illustrates a common characteristic that usually doesn't cause much problem until you reach the enlightening age of 40. Initially, pelvic tilt is the source of minor low back pain. If the hamstrings are weak, the stronger quadriceps (thigh muscles) tend to pull the pelvis forward. Also, as the belly slowly becomes more pronounced, greater stress to the low back is unavoidable. Like the domino effect, this tends to pull the shoulders forward, creating high stress on the neck. To compensate, the tendency is to change the gait, resulting in a "duck walk" pattern that strains the knees, legs, and so on. All as the result of a little overindulgence and laziness during our "invincible" younger years.

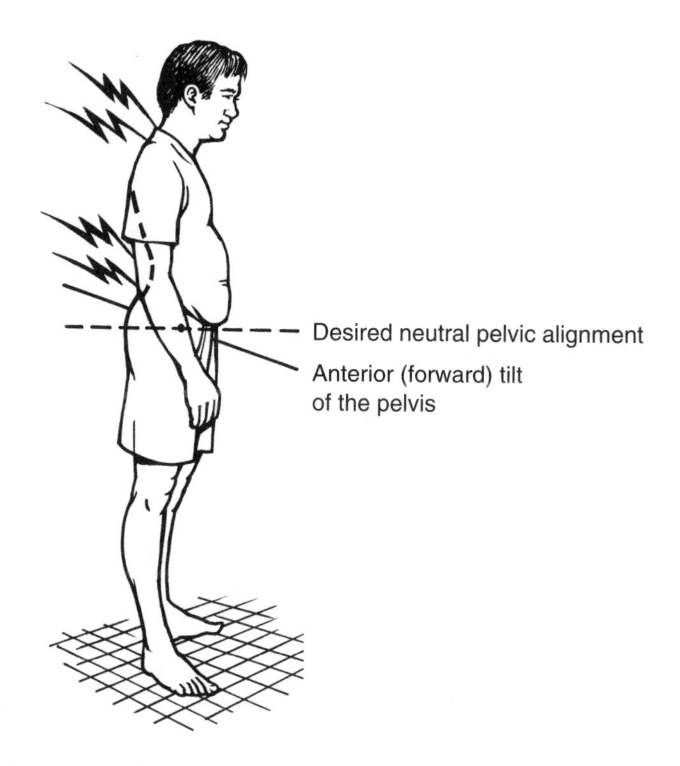

Posterior Pelvic Tilt

Another common postural ailment is the posterior tilt of the pelvis. Like the anterior example, a definite counterbalance effect begins to intensify if ignored. The head juts forward and the shoulders begin to

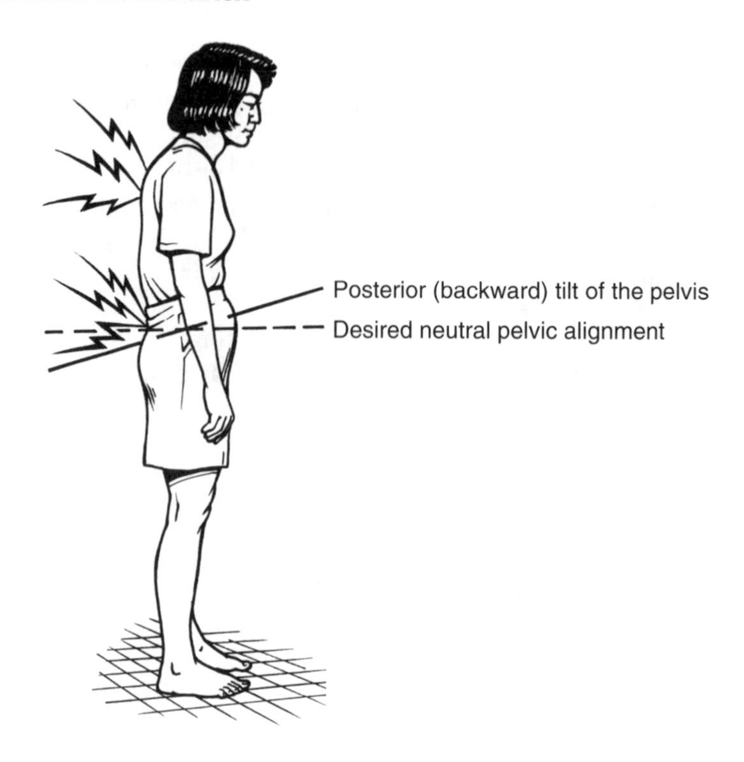

droop, placing stress on the upper back and neck. In effect, the muscles in the back have to take over for the skeletal system. This places tremendous force on the low back to compensate. (See above.)

So while the military posture that our parents so lovingly imposed on us is not entirely desirable, the alternative of forward or backward tilting pelvic girdles, drooping shoulders, and jutting heads is much more detrimental to our overall health and athletic potential.

Imbalance Problems

A weak core can certainly contribute to inefficient and extraneous movement patterns. These, in turn, can create muscle imbalances and structural dysfunction similar to the anterior and posterior pelvic tilts. For example, the baseball pitcher or tennis player are prime examples of athletes who develop one side much more than the other. A right-handed tennis player who has spent years honing his skills characteristically does all the necessary work with one side of the body. The right hand, forearm, upper arm, shoulder, leg, ankle, and foot end up doing the majority of the accelerating, decelerating, strengthening, and flexibility work. This muscular imbalance predisposes the athlete to almost certain posture problems.

Even the general population is inclined to favor a strong side when performing everyday tasks. Carrying the baby on one hip for several hours at a time, raking leaves with the same foot forward during every stroke, or routinely channel surfing with your dominate thumb can, over time, lead to serious misalignment. Old injuries left untreated, a bad pair of shoes, or that comfy old sofa eventually take their toll on you. If you have ever had a doctor, trainer, therapist, or chiropractor tell you that "one leg seems longer than the other" or "one shoulder is drooping," maybe your body's trying to tell you that something is structurally wrong.

Don't ignore pain: It's time to forget the antiquated concept of "playing through the pain." Subtle as the initial warnings may be, they should prompt you to determine the cause of the dysfunction and look for ways to eliminate it. Avoid the convenient "quick fix" of aspirin, taping, braces, and complete inactivity doctors commonly prescribe. Instead, begin at the core and work your way out. If you've avoided injury so far, following the plan we propose in this book increases your chances for continued health. Indeed, a well-developed core is the first step toward resolving structural problems and enhancing power transfer through efficient movement.

AUTOMATICITY

The ability to differentiate between one action and another, either in isolation or simultaneously, known as *automaticity*, is critically important to athletics. Even everyday activities such as driving require automaticity traits. Acute awareness while merging onto the highway during rush hour in the middle of a blizzard with hot coffee spilled onto your lap and kids fighting in the back seat can test the mettle of even the most experienced baby boomer.

You can approach even a basic task such as shooting a 15-foot jump shot in a way that enhances this differentiating ability. Simply make the task more difficult by requiring yourself to jump over a small barrier before shooting. After five minutes of this more demanding task, revert back to the normal 15-foot jump shot and see if your accuracy hasn't improved. This is a simple form of automaticity, whereby you challenge the system by bombarding it with additional variables to make a relatively easy task more challenging. The body learns to differentiate between one action and another, making movements more accurate and efficient. You have tremendous potential for discriminating among even the smallest stimuli, and it can be tapped through this kind of training. Many of the drills in this book contain an element of automaticity.

Basketball, like most sports, is dynamic, in that players must keep their feet in constant motion. While a base of support is important in all sports, it is certainly not the primary stabilization factor. Unlike sumo wrestlers, basketball players rarely have the luxury of standing in one spot with their feet firmly planted on the floor. Consequently, sumo wrestlers derive most of their postural control from their stable base of support on the ground, while basketball players get their stabilization primarily from the core. Pat Riley, head coach of the Miami Heat and former head coach of the New York Knicks, enthusiastically embraces the concept of increasing stabilization through training for automaticity and, as a result, has taken it to the extreme. Thus the Knicks have incorporated such equipment as *balance boards* and *hard foam rollers* into many aspects of their training to make tasks more complex and to intensify trunk stabilization through continuous motion. (See photos below and on page 71.)

We advise caution, however: From a safety standpoint, many of these exercises pose a higher than normal risk of injury. Whether you're an athlete or a weekend warrior, we recommend that you first consult a professional trainer or coach who has experience and understanding of this mode of training.

THE EXERCISES

Trunk stabilization exercises are intended to challenge your senses. You will begin to discriminate between subtle changes in your body's equilibrium, automatically adjusting to those changes in a conservative—

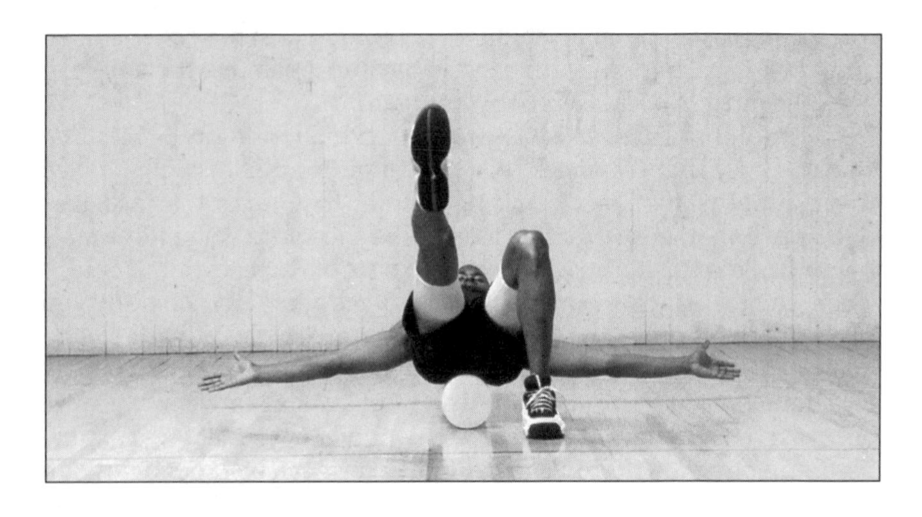

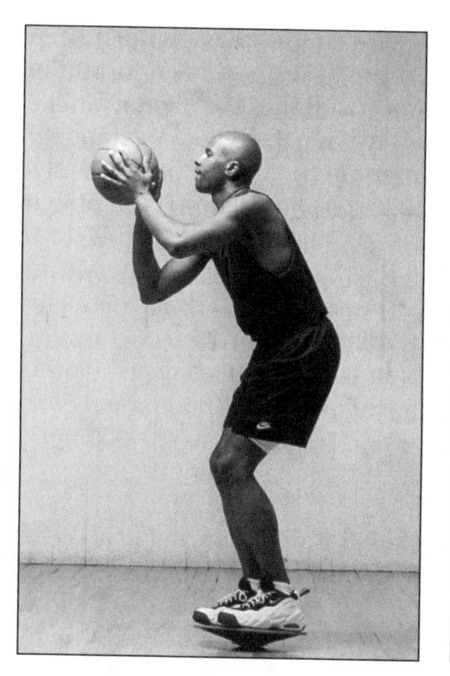

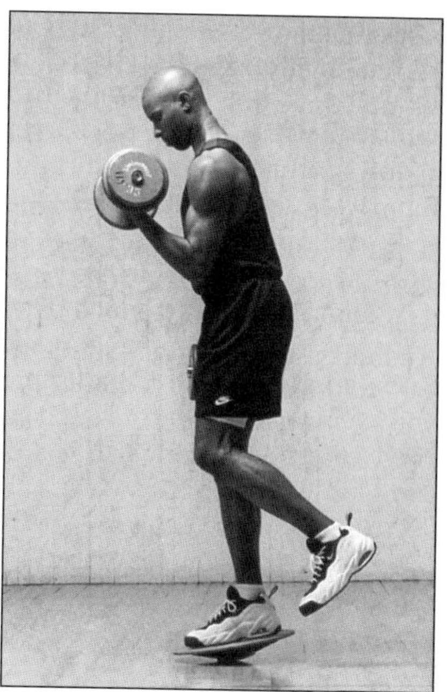

yet effective—effort. Certainly, the goal is *not* to structurally develop the abdominals to generate greater force and power or to augment your emerging washboard abs. Don't make the common mistake of applying too much force instead of using moderately sufficient force more effectively. Too much force tends to detract from the intended purpose of the action.

For example, accuracy would definitely be sacrificed in lieu of added force if you took a full windup prior to throwing a dart. Recognize that applied force and increased sensitivity of motion will progressively enhance stabilization, accuracy of movement, and efficient power transfer.

Most of the exercises outlined in the later chapters of this book contribute to the development of balance and help to promote correct posture. The exercises presented in this chapter, however, were designed to specifically encourage basic trunk and torso stabilization. These exercises are a safe and effective way of reinforcing the elements of good posture through a wide range of movement. We'll revisit some of them in later chapters as well.

In some of the exercises, we'll make a simple action such as sitting more complex by requiring you to perform the task on apparatus such as a large TheraBall. Now the sedentary action of sitting becomes dynamic. This triggers your posture-maintaining muscles to work to maintain balance. Eventually, you'll make these adjustments automatically as your sensory mechanisms learn to do the job of maintaining equilibrium for you. Postural awareness, spine alignment, coordination, muscular balance, muscular toning, and sensory mechanisms can all be improved simply by sitting on a large ball.

For more information contact the San Francisco Spine Institute at Seton Medical Center in San Francisco, CA 650-985-7500 and request their *Dynamic Lumbar Stabilization Program*. To secure a TheraBall (also referred to as a Bodyball, Gymnic, Physioball, or Physio/Gymnic) contact SporTime in Atlanta, GA 800-444-5700, or The Saunders Group, Inc. of Chaska, MN 800-456-1289.

Exercise Guidelines and Preparation

Adhere to the following guidelines to help ensure safe progress:

- Receive clearance from your doctor prior to initiating any new program.
- Make sure equipment is clean, undamaged, and maintained to meet the manufacturer's standards.
- Use spotters whenever possible.
- Emphasize precise technique over advancing to greater sets, reps, or more difficult exercises.
- Understand the purpose of each exercise.
- Perform each exercise slowly.

Before you begin, try some *isolated* and *co-contractions* of the core muscles to help you find your *neutral* position. Stand tall with your hands on your hips and simultaneously contract the abdominals and low back muscles, developing a "feel" for the muscles involved. If you look at yourself in a mirror, you should see a relatively straight line between your ear, shoulder, hip, knee, and ankle. The straight line should be natural, not forced (no need to salute the flag). Now, relax the abdominals just enough to allow the tension from the low back muscles to tilt the pelvis forward. See how well you can control this action. Once again, contract the abdominals and low back muscles (neutral position) simultaneously. This time relax the low back muscles, allowing the abdominals to pull at their low attachment, and slowly tilt the pelvis back. Understanding the function of the muscles involved is important from the standpoint of total trunk stabilization. Initially, you will have to make an effort to apply this newfound control to the following exercises. As you become proficient, you won't have to make a conscious effort to maintain the neutral position.

Trunk Stabilization Exercises

Low Back Isolate (Bridging)

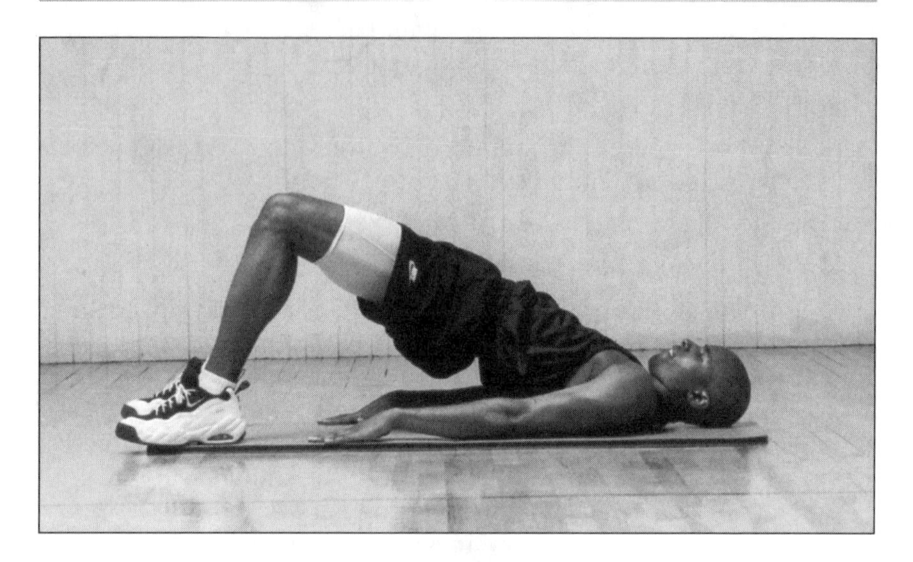

Slow

PREPARATION

- Lie on the floor with entire spine in contact with the floor.
- Flex knees to 90 degrees.
- Place feet flat on the floor, shoulder-width apart.
- Place hands on the floor, next to the hips. (Keep the hands off the floor as balance improves.)

ACTION

- Contract the low back muscles and gluteals and lift the hips off the floor.
- Keep the shoulders and upper back in contact with the floor.
- Keep body weight off the neck.
- Hold for 5 to 10 seconds.
- Return to the starting position.
- Immediately repeat.

Note: Place a pillow under the head and neck for added comfort and support.

Low Back Isolate (Bridging) With Leg Extension

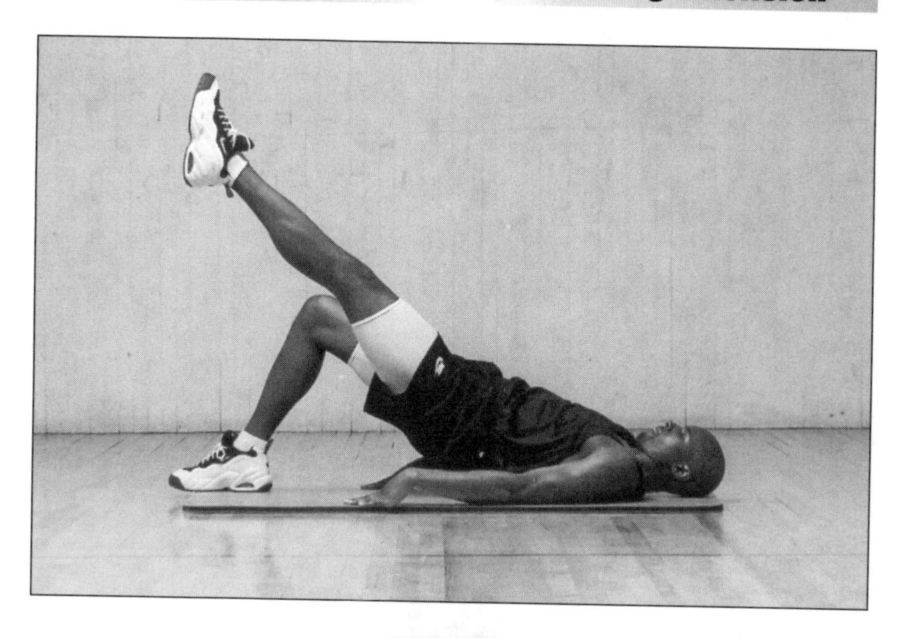

Slow

PREPARATION

- Lie on the floor with entire spine in contact with the floor.
- Flex knees to 90 degrees.
- Place feet flat on the floor, shoulder-width apart.
- Place hands on the floor, next to the hips. (Keep the hands off the floor as balance improves.)

ACTION

- Contract the low back muscles and gluteals and lift the hips off the floor.
- Keep the shoulders and upper back in contact with the floor.
- Keep body weight off the neck.
- Extend the left leg at about 45 degrees to the floor.
- Hold for 5 to 10 seconds.
- Return to the starting position.
- Immediately repeat.
- Continue on the same side for one complete set or alternate reps with the opposite side.

Note: Place a pillow under the head and neck for added comfort and support.

Foot Squeeze

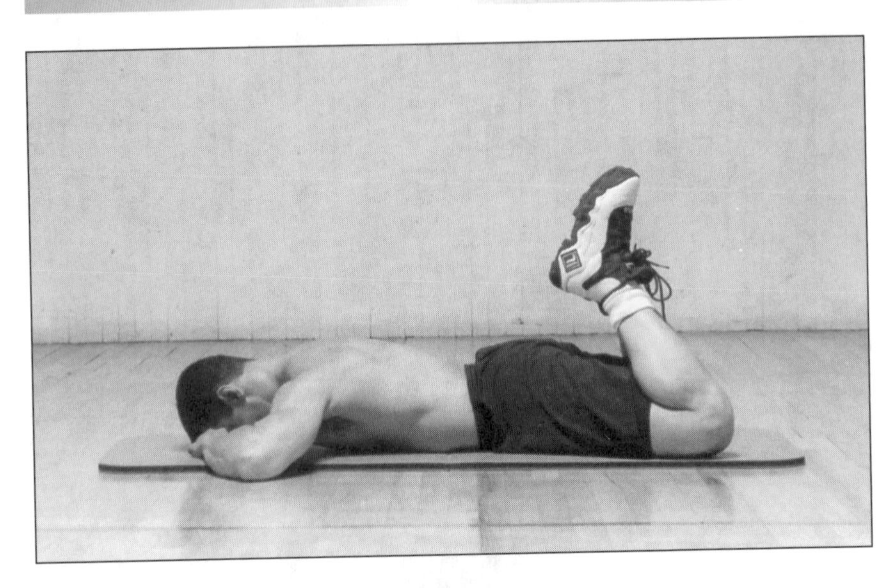

Slow

PREPARATION

- Lie on the floor on your stomach.
- Keep knees shoulder-width apart and flex to 90 degrees.
- Touch heels together.
- Rest forehead or chin on hands.

ACTION

- Contract the abdominals and low back muscles simultaneously.
- Squeeze the heels together using the gluteals and adductors (the inner thigh muscles).
- Hold for 5 to 10 seconds.
- Return to the starting position.
- Immediately repeat.

Note: Place a pillow under the hips for added comfort and support.

Hip Internal and External Rotation

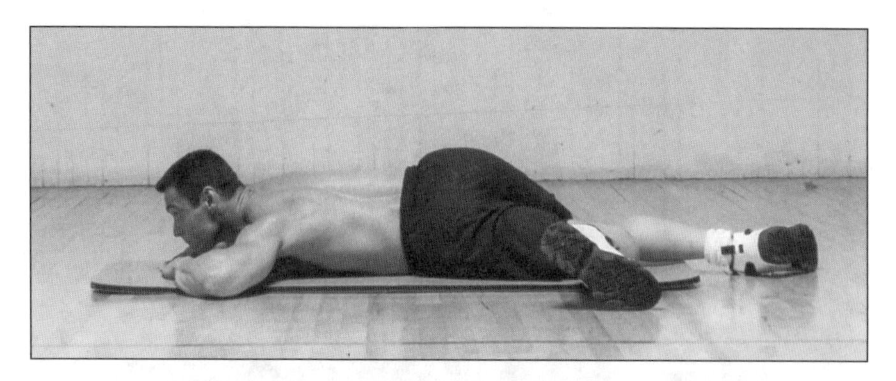

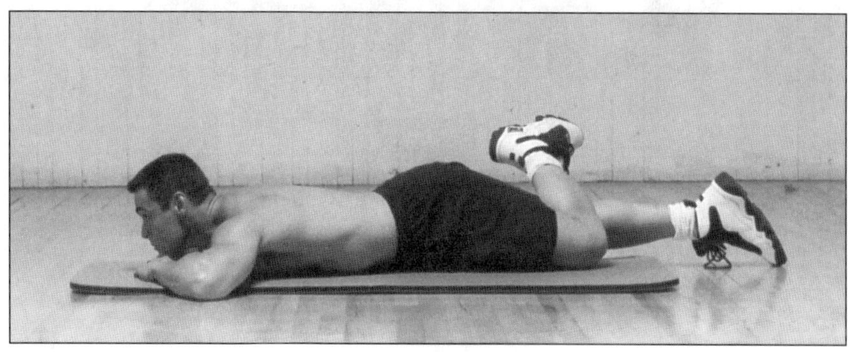

Slow

PREPARATION

- Lie on the floor on stomach.
- Keep knees shoulder-width apart.
- Extend right leg.
- Flex left knee to 90 degrees.
- Rest forehead or chin on hands.

ACTION

- Contract the abdominal and low back muscles simultaneously.
- Drop the left leg to the left as far as possible without the opposite (right) hip rising off the floor.
- Bring the left leg back to the starting position and immediately drop to the right side. Again, do not allow the opposite (right) hip to lift off the floor.
- Immediately repeat.

Note: Don't allow the leg to just flop side to side. Control the movement with the pelvic muscles. Place a pillow under the hips for added comfort and support.

Superman

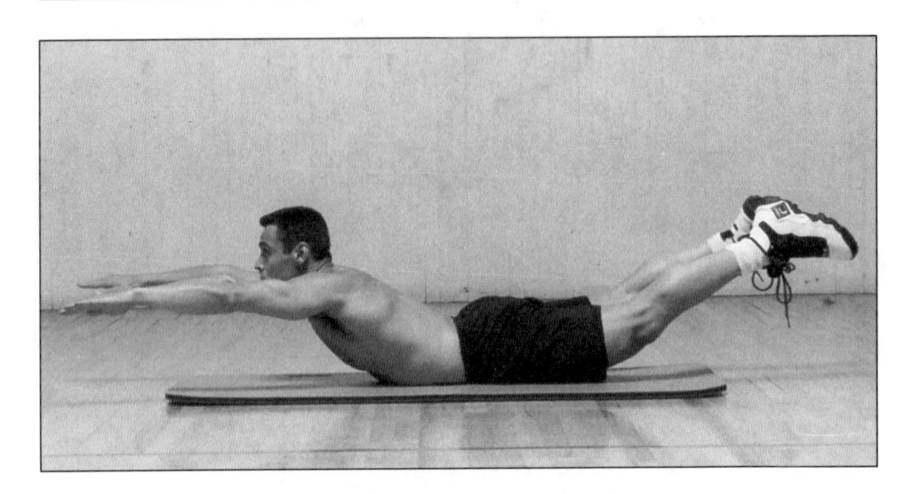

Slow

PREPARATION

- Lie on the floor on stomach.
- Extend arms overhead.

ACTION

- Simultaneously lift the upper body and the legs off the floor.
- Hold the contracted position for 3 to 5 seconds.
- Return to the starting position.
- Immediately repeat.

Note: Chapter 6 details several variations of this exercise.

Hip Extension

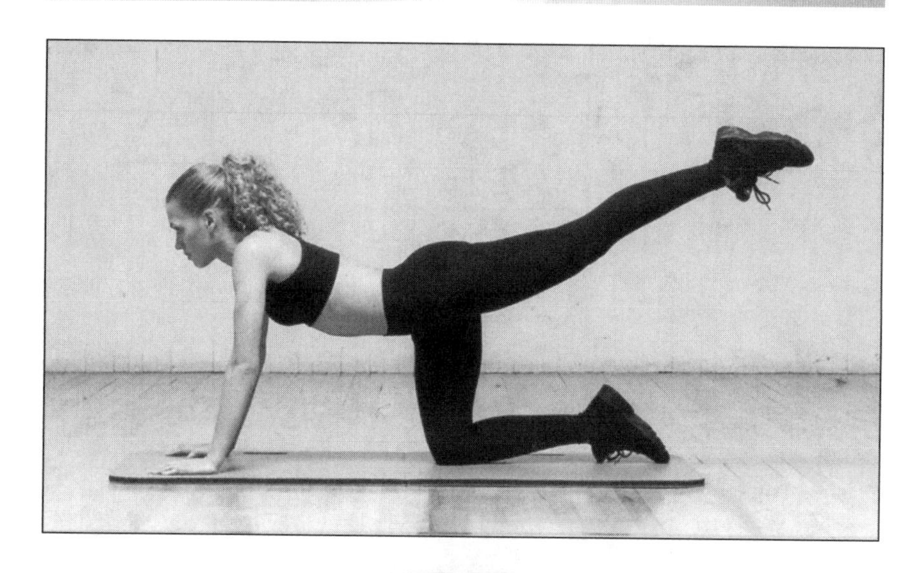

Slow

PREPARATION

- Place hands and right knee on the floor.
- Extend the left leg, touching the floor with the left toes.
- Lift head slightly.

ACTION

- Contract the left gluteal and hamstring, lifting the leg as high as comfortably possible.
- Hold for one count (i.e., "one-thousand-one").
- Return to the starting position.
- Continue on the same side for one set.
- Repeat on the opposite side.

Note: You can perform this exercise from a standing position. Place the hands against a wall and follow the *action* directions listed above. In addition, chapter 6 details several variations of this exercise.

Four-Point Forward Lean

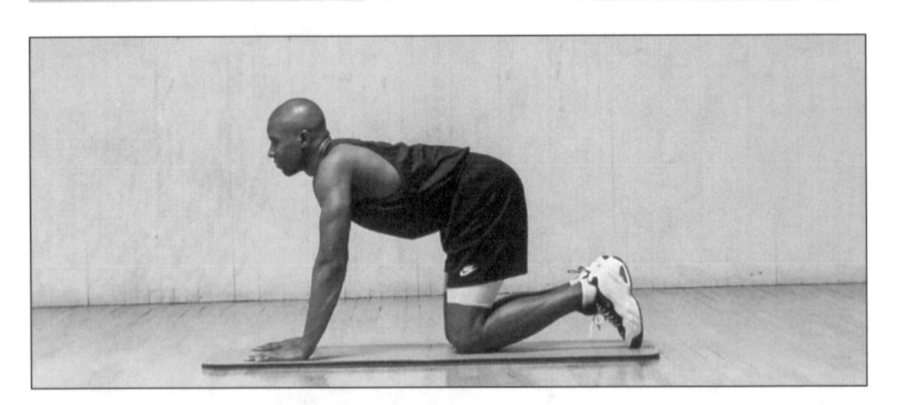

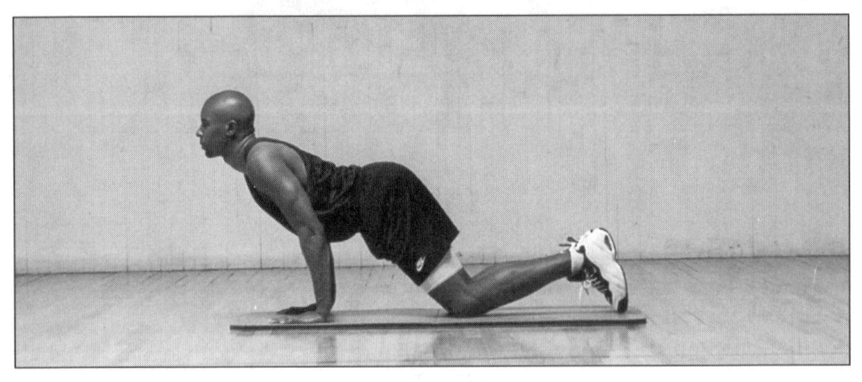

Slow

PREPARATION

- Place both hands and knees on the floor with arms and upper thighs at a 90-degree angle to the floor. (As strength and balance improve, move the hands to a starting position slightly ahead of the shoulders, more in line with the top of the head.)
- Keep back straight.
- Lift head slightly.

ACTION

- Contract the abdominal and low back muscles simultaneously.
- Lean forward so that most of the upper body weight is over the hands.
- Hold for several seconds.
- Return to the starting position.
- Immediately repeat.

TheraBall Neutral Position

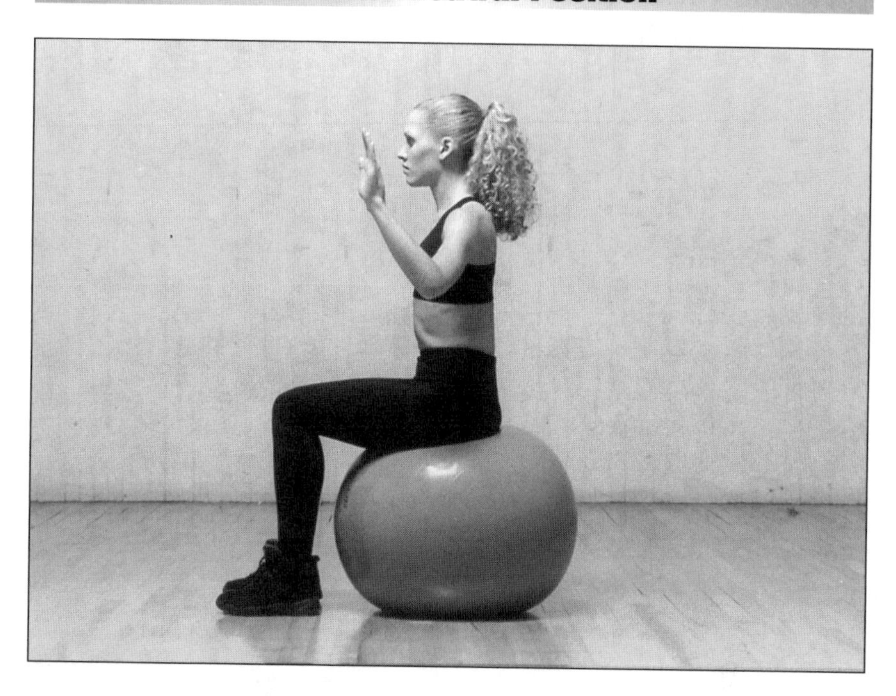

PREPARATION/ACTION

- Inflate ball according to the manufacturer's specifications.
- Choose the appropriate ball size: When seated, upper thigh should be parallel to the ground or slightly higher.
- Place feet flat on the floor.
- Establish the neutral position by contracting the abdominals and low back muscles simultaneously.
- Keep back straight.
- Hold hands up in the ready position.

TheraBall Sitting Position: Anterior and Posterior Tilt

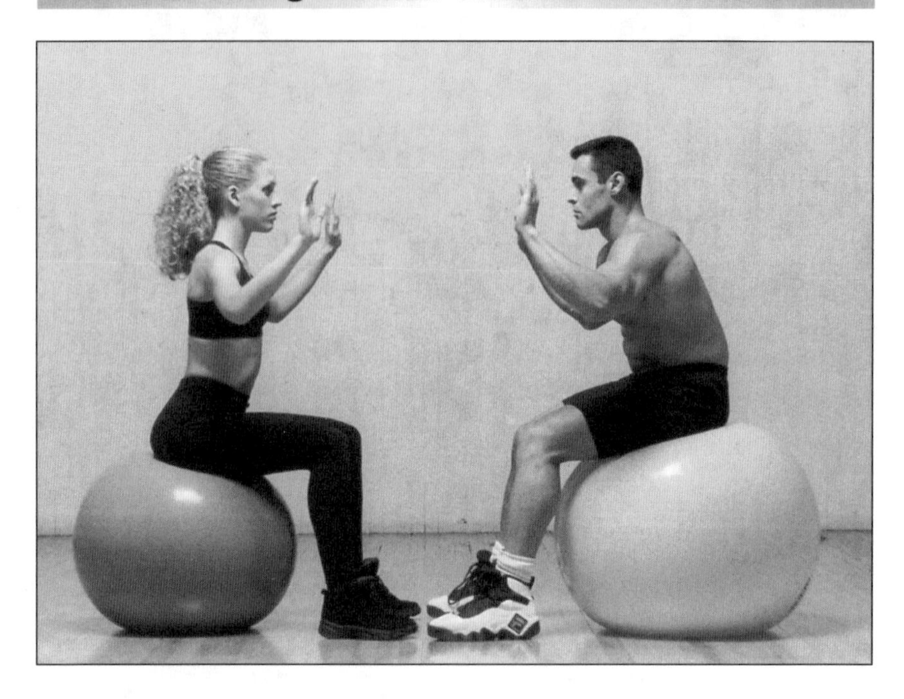

PREPARATION

- Inflate ball according to manufacturer's specifications.
- Choose the appropriate ball size: When seated, upper thigh should be parallel to the ground or slightly higher.
- Place feet flat on the floor.
- Establish the neutral position by contracting the abdominals and low back muscles simultaneously (see photo on page 81).
- Keep back straight.
- Hold hands up in the ready position.

ACTION

- In a slow and controlled manner, relax the abdominals, creating a forward tilt of the pelvis (the buttocks will roll slightly over the ball).
- Return to the neutral position.
- Allow the low back muscles to relax slightly, thereby tilting the pelvis backward.
- Continue forward and backward tilts for 30 to 60 seconds.
- Do several sets.

TheraBall Sitting Position: Lateral Tilt

Slow

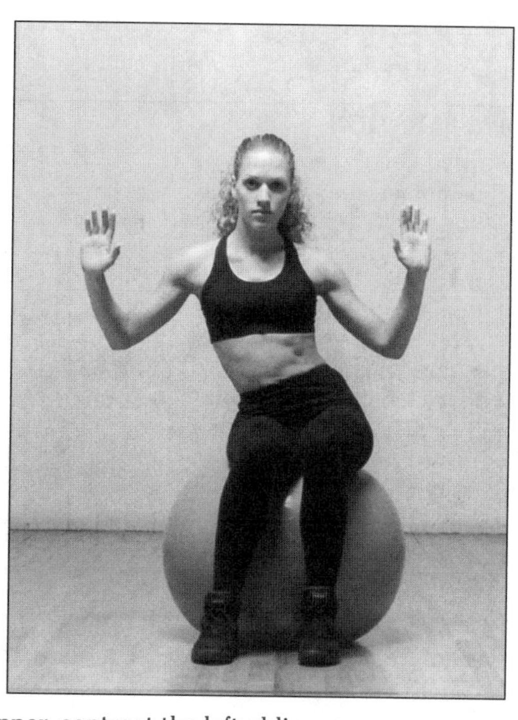

PREPARATION

- Inflate ball according to manufacturer's specifications.
- Choose the appropriate ball size: When seated, upper thigh should be parallel to the ground or slightly higher.
- Place feet flat on the floor.
- Establish the neutral position by contracting the abdominals and low back muscles simultaneously (see photo on page 81).
- Keep back straight.
- Hold hands up in the ready position.

ACTION

- In a slow and controlled manner, contract the left obliques.
- Return to the neutral position.
- Immediately repeat on the opposite side.
- Continue lateral tilts for 30 to 60 seconds.
- Do several sets.

TheraBall Sitting Position With Hip Rotation

Slow

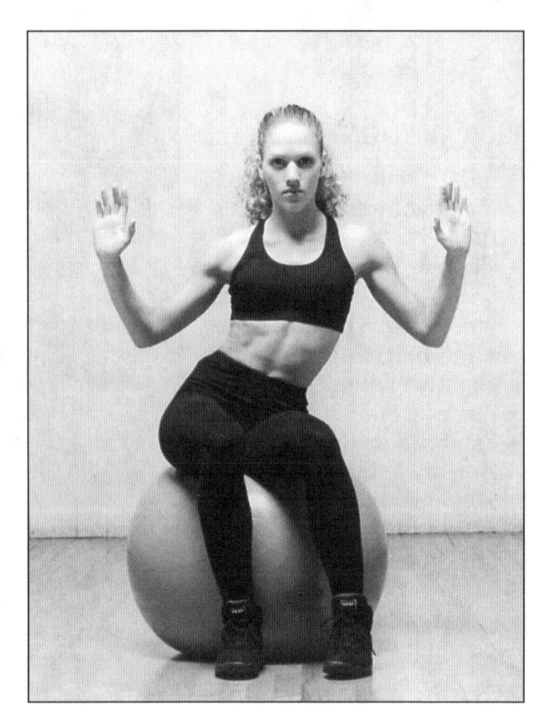

PREPARATION

- Inflate ball according to manufacturer's specifications.
- Choose the appropriate ball size: When seated, upper thigh should be parallel to the ground or slightly higher.
- Place feet flat on the floor.
- Establish the neutral position by contracting the abdominals and low back muscles simultaneously (see photo on page 81).
- Keep back straight.
- Hold hands up in the ready position.

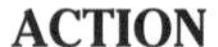

ACTION

- In a slow and controlled manner, begin rotating the hips only, keeping the head and upper torso stationary.
- Rotate clockwise for 10 to 20 revolutions.
- Repeat in the opposite direction.

TheraBall Sitting Position: Leg Extension

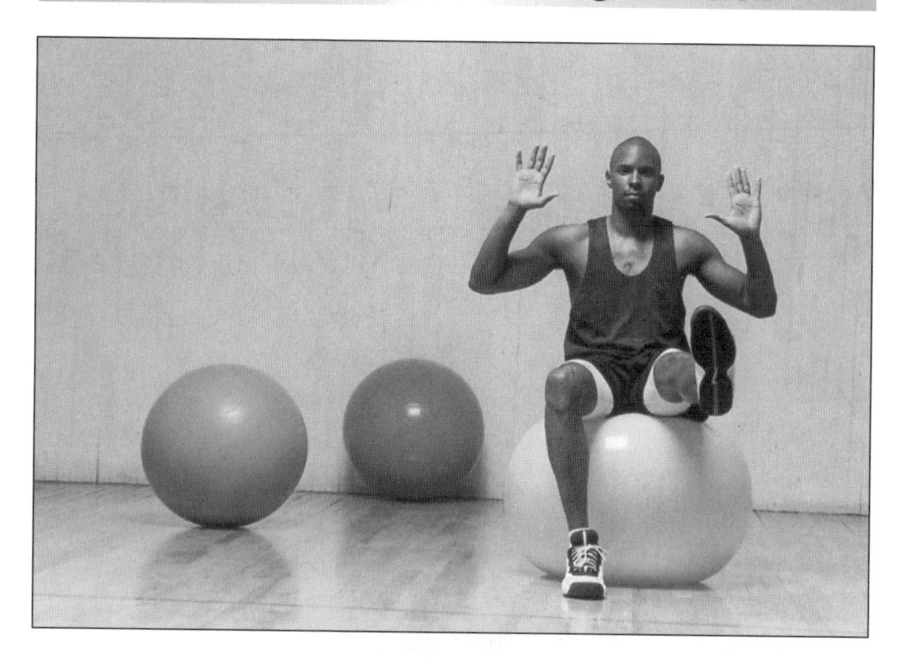

Slow

PREPARATION

- Inflate ball according to manufacturer's specifications.
- Choose the appropriate ball size: When seated, upper thigh should be parallel to the ground or slightly higher.
- Place feet flat on the floor.
- Establish the neutral position by contracting the abdominals and low back muscles simultaneously (see photo on page 81).
- Keep back straight.
- Hold hands up in the ready position.

ACTION

- Slowly extend the left leg to a position approximately horizontal to the ground.
- Hold for 5 to 10 seconds.
- Return to the neutral position.
- Continue on the same side for one complete set or alternate reps with the opposite side.

TheraBall Sitting Position: 45-Degree Leg Extension

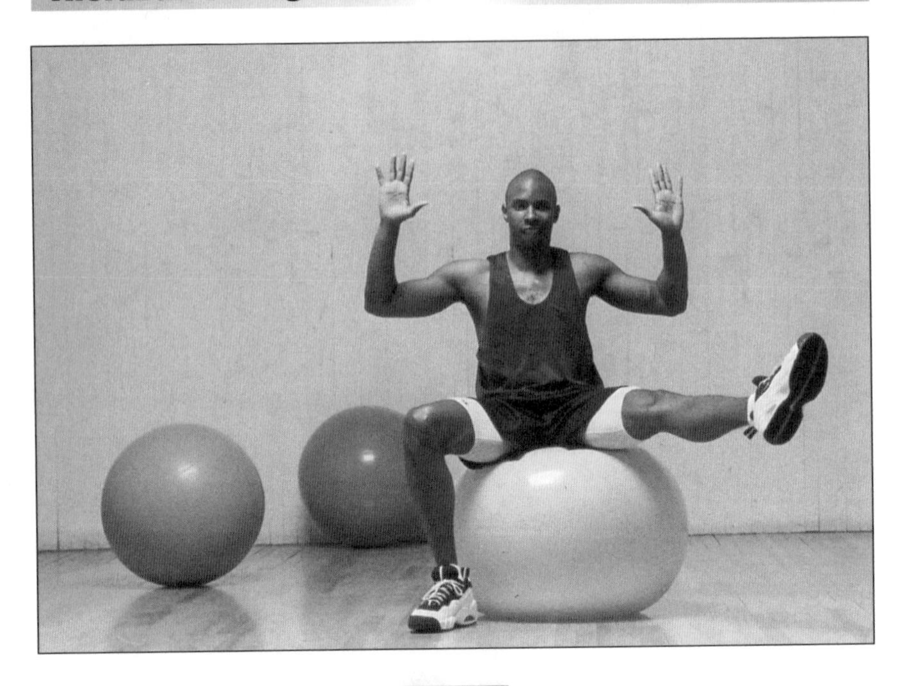

Slow

PREPARATION

- Inflate ball according to manufacturer's specifications.
- Choose the appropriate ball size: When seated, upper thigh should be parallel to the ground or slightly higher.
- Place feet flat on the floor.
- Establish the neutral position by contracting the abdominals and low back muscles simultaneously (see photo on page 81).
- Keep back straight.
- Hold hands up in the ready position.

ACTION

- Slowly extend the left leg at a 45-degree angle, approximately horizontal to the ground.
- Hold for 5 to 10 seconds.
- Return to the neutral position.
- Continue on the same side for one complete set or alternate reps with the opposite side.

TheraBall Supine Roller

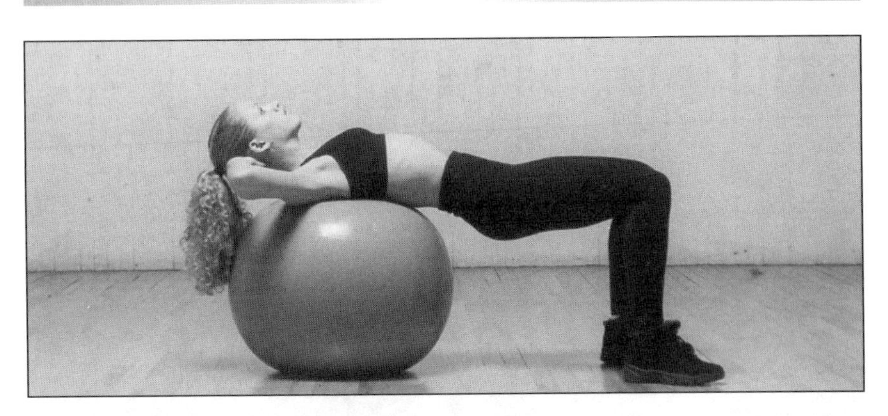

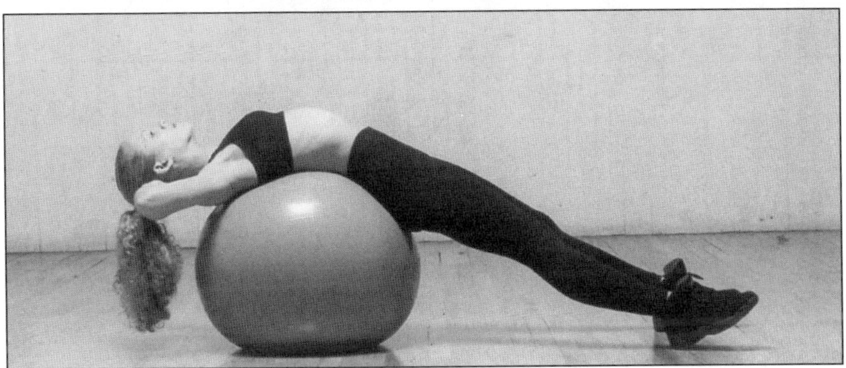

Slow

PREPARATION

- Inflate ball according to manufacturer's specifications.
- Choose the appropriate ball size.
- Position shoulder blades on top of the ball.
- Keep torso and thighs relatively straight throughout the exercise.
- Flex knees to 90 degrees.
- Place feet flat on the floor.
- Establish the neutral position by contracting the abdominals and low back muscles simultaneously.
- Place hands behind the head. (If balance is a problem, spread your arms out to your sides.)

ACTION

- Slowly push and extend with both legs.
- The ball should roll down the spine to the small of the back.
- Hold for 5 to 10 seconds.
- Pull with the legs to return to the starting position.
- Immediately repeat.

TheraBall Supine Full Body Extension

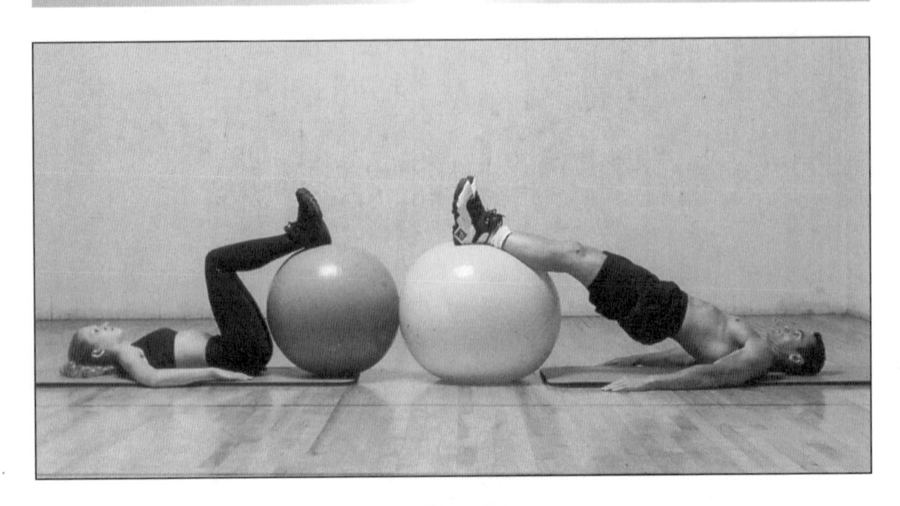

Slow

PREPARATION

- Inflate ball according to manufacturer's specifications.
- Choose the appropriate ball size.
- Lie on the floor with entire spine in contact with the floor.
- Flex knees and hips to 90 degrees.
- Place heels on top of ball.
- Position hands next to the hips, flat on the floor.

ACTION

- Slowly extend with both legs (the ball will roll).
- Keep the abdominals and low back muscles tight throughout the exercise.
- Avoid inordinate pressure on the head and neck.
- Hold for 5 to 10 seconds.
- Slowly return to the starting position.
- Immediately repeat.

Note: Place a pillow under the head and neck for added comfort and support.

TheraBall Prone Wobble

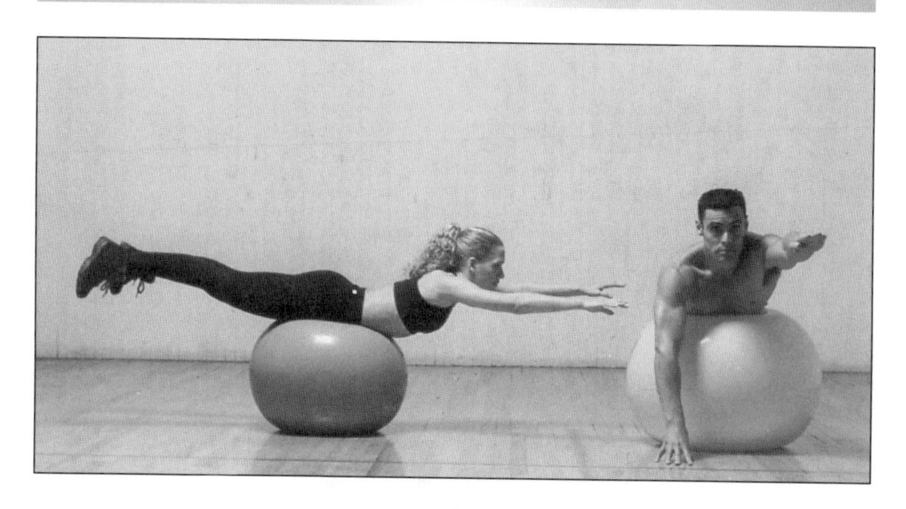

Slow

PREPARATION

- Lie on stomach on a smaller ball.
- Place hands and feet on floor.

ACTION

- Experiment with different "superman" positions (e.g., one hand off the floor, both hands off the floor, one foot, both feet, extend one arm and one leg, extend both arms and both legs, and so on).

Note: If the pressure on your stomach is uncomfortable, stop.

6

Ab Fitness Exercises

The abdominal and low back exercises to follow are better suited for the novice fitness enthusiast but will also serve as the nucleus of exercises for athletes at every level. Advance from this fitness level to the more demanding ab strength exercises only after mastering the exercises described here. If, after completing the 24-week fitness program described in chapter 9, you feel your technique meets the standards set in the descriptions, you're ready to move up to the next level.

Remember, technique is much more important than additional repetitions or added resistance. If you prefer to stay at the ab fitness level, by all means do so. More is not always better. Many of our elite athletes are perfectly content to stay with the ab fitness program for as long as they continue to see positive physical changes. As we discussed in chapter 4, you may reach a point at which you are content with your strength level, functional capacity, and the appearance of your trunk and torso. If this happens, you can switch to a maintenance program in which intensity remains high but the frequency and duration of your workouts can drop considerably. We'll discuss this further in chapter 9.

If you have been inactive for a long time, you can expect some minor muscle soreness a day or two after you start the program. This slight discomfort is a signal that your body is responding to a positive exercise stimulus. If the pain becomes chronic and continues into the second week, review your exercise technique and consult a health professional to determine the cause. Understand that the pain may vary from day to day and from person to person. Any time you introduce a new exercise, routine, intensity, or number of reps, your body will respond differently.

Whatever your reason for initiating an exercise regimen, make a firm vow to stick with it, especially during the initial weeks. Don't be in a hurry. While "waking one morning to discover that you're out of shape" is a common experience, we can assure you that in most cases loss of fitness occurs gradually over many years. So don't count on an instant transformation back to those youthful years. We guarantee that you will see noticeable improvement if you maintain a disciplined program such as the one outlined in chapter 9.

If, however, you limit your routine strictly to the core region, you will not adequately improve the other components of health and fitness. The abdominal and low back routines that we suggest here must be part of a complete program that includes the fitness variables of

- total body muscular strength,
- total body muscular endurance,
- cardiorespiratory efficiency,
- body composition, and
- flexibility.

Set realistic, attainable goals. Recognize that slow progress is still progress. While daily transformation might seem undetectable, incrementally, these changes begin to add up. Over time you will definitely see results. Can you handle the commitment? It will require a change in lifestyle. For starters, we suggest that you keep a daily record. This will serve the dual role of indicating progress and maintaining motivation. Another good motivational tool is to train with a partner. The partner can help spot, deliver feedback concerning proper technique, and provide encouragement.

Let's get started!

Ab and Low Back Fitness Exercises

Straight-Leg Side Crunch

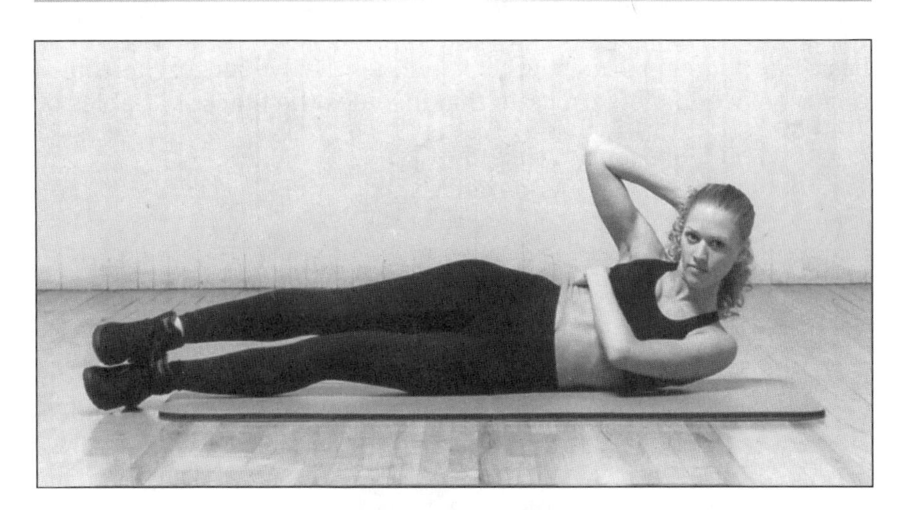

Ab Fitness (Obliques)
Slow

PREPARATION

- Lie on the left side.
- Keep legs straight.
- Place right hand behind the head.
- Place left hand on the working obliques.

ACTION

- Slowly contract the right internal and external obliques and lift the shoulder two to six inches off the floor.
- Hold for one count (i.e., "one-thousand-one").
- Return to the starting position.
- Immediately begin the next repetition (do not relax the obliques between reps).
- Continue on the same side for one set.
- Repeat on the opposite side.

Note: If you are having difficulty successfully accomplishing the movement, "hook" your feet under a sofa, chair, or partner to increase leverage. Do not drop the shoulders and buttocks back toward the floor. In this position, the stronger rectus abdominis (upper ab) muscles will do most of the work. As with all drills, never allow the abdominals to relax between repetitions.

Straight-Leg Side Crunch With Leg Lift

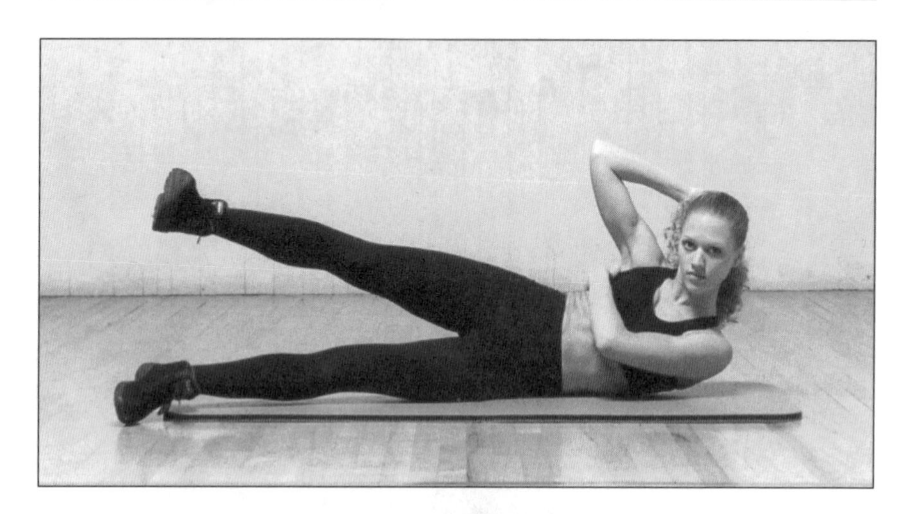

Ab Fitness (Obliques)
Slow

PREPARATION

- Lie on the left side.
- Keep legs straight.
- Place right hand behind the head.
- Place left hand on the working obliques.

ACTION

- Slowly contract the right internal and external obliques while simultaneously lifting the right leg.
- Lift shoulder two to six inches while lifting the right foot about one to two feet off the floor.
- Hold for one count.
- Return to the starting position.
- Immediately repeat.
- Continue on the same side for one set.
- Repeat on the opposite side.

Note: If you are ready for a greater challenge, lift both legs off the floor, still making sure you stay positioned on your side. Do not drop your shoulders and buttocks back toward the floor.

Bent-Knee Side Raise

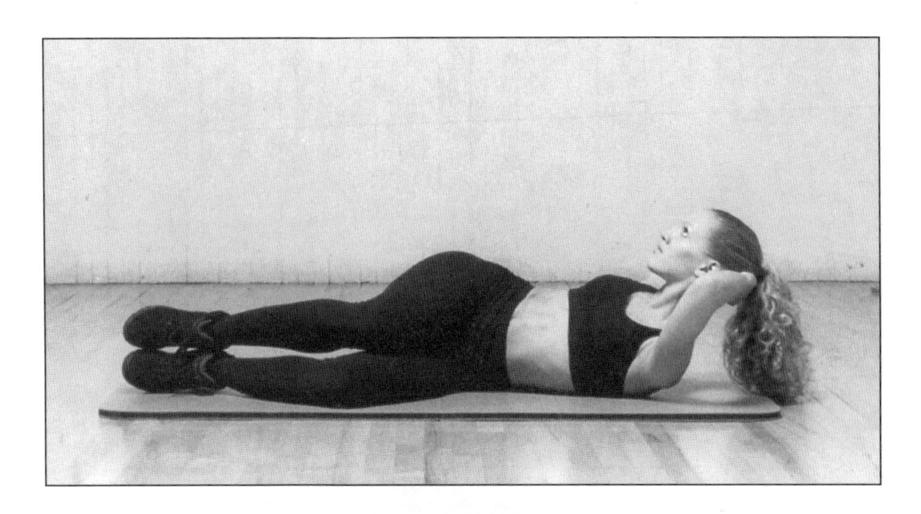

Ab Fitness (Obliques)
Slow

PREPARATION

- Lie on the left hip.
- Flex knees to 90 degrees.
- Focus eyes on ceiling.
- Keep shoulders square, both elbows "flat" to the floor.
- Place hands behind the head.

ACTION

- Contract the obliques and slowly lift (do not curl) the shoulders to a position two to six inches off the floor.
- Hold for one count.
- Return to the starting position.
- Immediately repeat.
- Continue on the same side for one set.
- Repeat on the opposite side.

Note: To vary the intensity, experiment with different arm positions, such as

- keep arms straight and reach toward the feet, and
- fold arms across the chest.

The Squirm

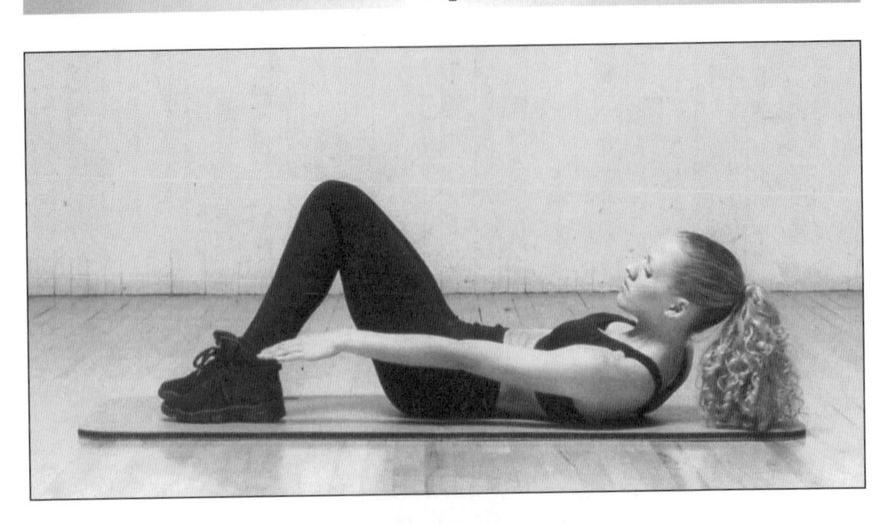

Ab Fitness (Obliques)
Slow

PREPARATION

- Lie on back with knees flexed and back straight.
- Place feet flat on the floor, approximately 12 inches from the buttocks.
- Keep arms at sides, resting on the floor.
- Tuck chin to the chest.
- Touch shoulder blades to the floor or raise slightly (one to two inches).

ACTION

- Squeeze the obliques and reach and tap the left foot with the left hand.
- Alternate sides.

Note: To make the exercise more challenging, *isometrically* hold each repetition for three to five seconds. (An isometric contraction is one in which there is no lengthening or shortening of the muscle fibers. You simply hold one position for a few seconds.)

The Advanced Squirm

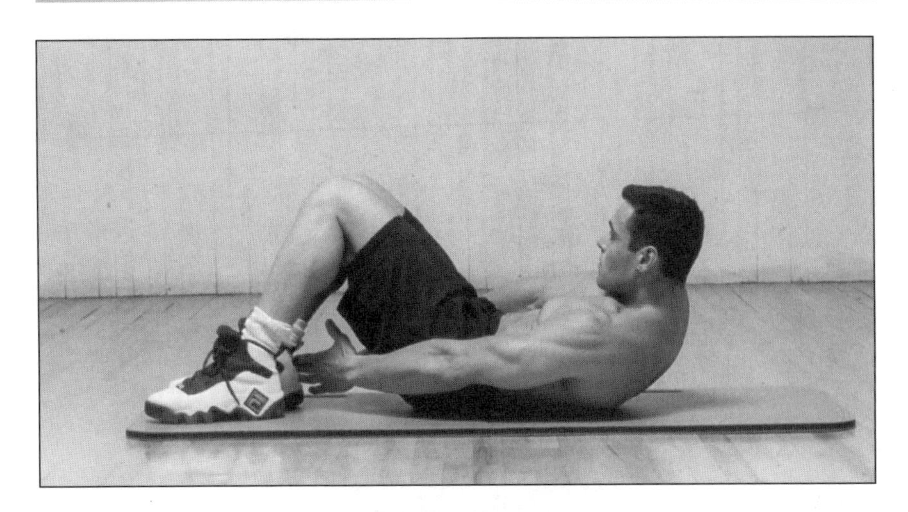

Ab Fitness (Obliques)
Moderate

PREPARATION

- Lie on back with knees flexed and back straight.
- Place feet flat on the floor, approximately 12 inches from the buttocks.
- Raise shoulders 8 to 12 inches off the floor, holding this position for the duration of the set.
- Keep arms at sides, resting on the floor.
- Tuck chin to the chest.

ACTION

- With the shoulders in the up position, reach the left hand under the legs to the right foot.
- Alternate sides.

Crossed-Leg Oblique Crunch

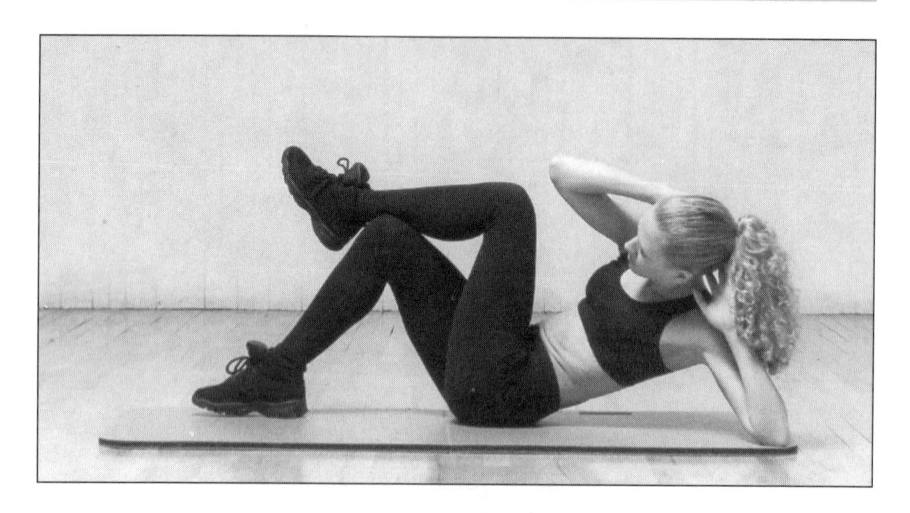

Ab Fitness (Obliques)
Slow

PREPARATION

- Lie on back.
- Flex right knee to 90 degrees, placing the right foot flat on the floor.
- Cross the left leg over the right.
- Place hands behind the head, keeping shoulders on the floor.
- Keep the left elbow in contact with the floor throughout the set.

ACTION

- Using the left elbow for leverage, "crunch" the obliques by raising the right elbow and tap the left knee.
- Hold for one count.
- Return to the starting position.
- Continue toward the same side for one set.
- Repeat on the opposite side.

Note: For a greater challenge, rest the left knee on the right knee. For a less difficult exercise, rest the left ankle on the right knee.

Advanced Crossed-Leg Oblique Crunch

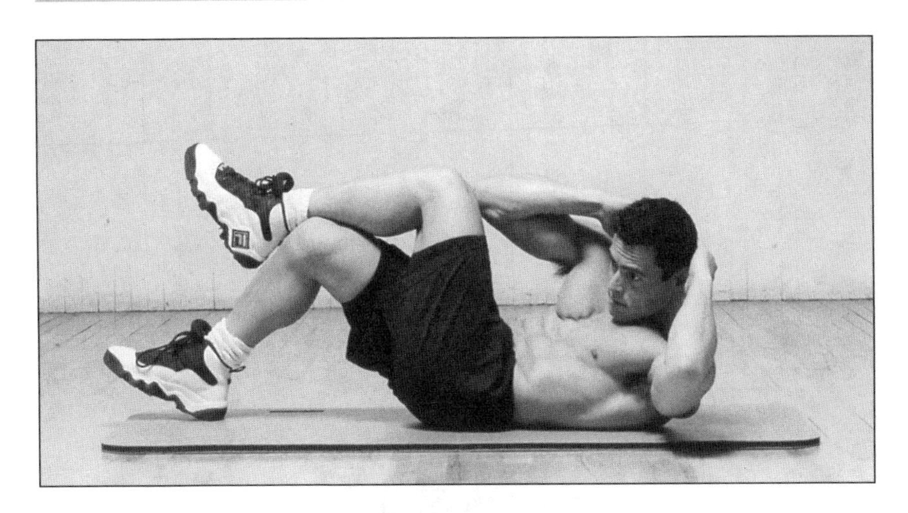

Ab Fitness (Obliques)
Slow

PREPARATION

- Lie on back, keeping back straight.
- Flex right knee 90 degrees, placing the right foot flat on the floor.
- Cross the left leg over the right.
- Place hands behind the head.

ACTION

- Lift both shoulder blades off the floor and twist so that the right elbow taps the *top* of the left knee.
- Hold for one count.
- Return to the starting position.
- Continue on the same side until you finish the set.
- Repeat on the opposite side.

Note: For a greater challenge, rest the left knee on the right knee. For a less difficult exercise, rest the left ankle on the right knee. *Never* pull on the head or neck to assist in the movement. As with all drills, never allow the abdominals to relax between repetitions.

Butterfly Curl-Up With Alternating Twist

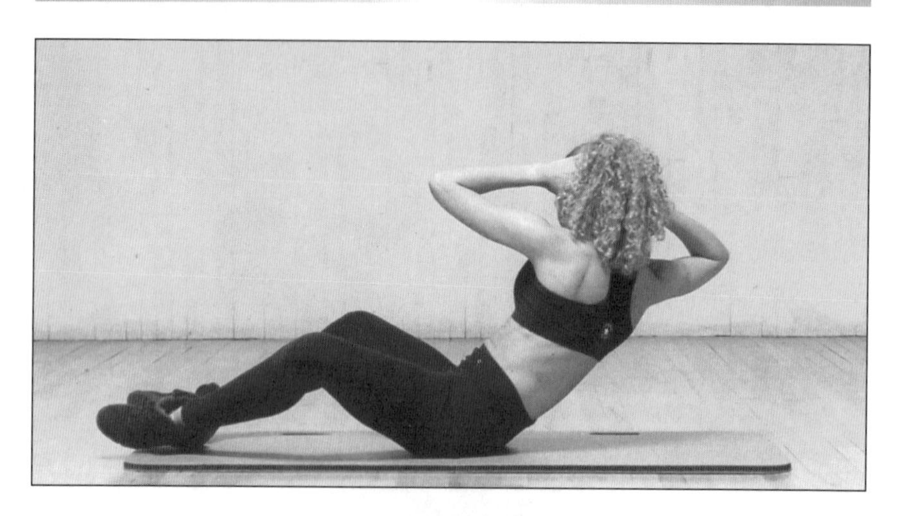

Ab Fitness (Obliques)
Slow

PREPARATION

- Lie on back.
- Place soles of the feet together, as close to the buttocks as possible. The closer the feet are to the buttocks, the more difficult the exercise.
- Drop knees to the sides into the "butterfly" position.
- Tilt head back, focusing eyes on the ceiling.
- Place hands behind the head.

ACTION

- Lift the shoulder blades off the floor and twist the upper torso and elbow toward the opposite knee.
- Return to the starting position.
- Repeat toward the *alternate* side (right side then left side equals one repetition).

Note: Experiment with different arm positions to vary the difficulty of this and other exercises. Start with arms extended and reach between the legs. As strength levels improve, fold the arms across the chest, then advance to putting them behind the head. As you continue to grow stronger, raise the upper body and touch the elbow to the knee. You can change the positions of the legs and feet (extended or up close to the buttocks) to make the movement easier or more difficult. Hooking the feet can be of great help to the beginner.

Butterfly Curl-Up With Continuous Twist

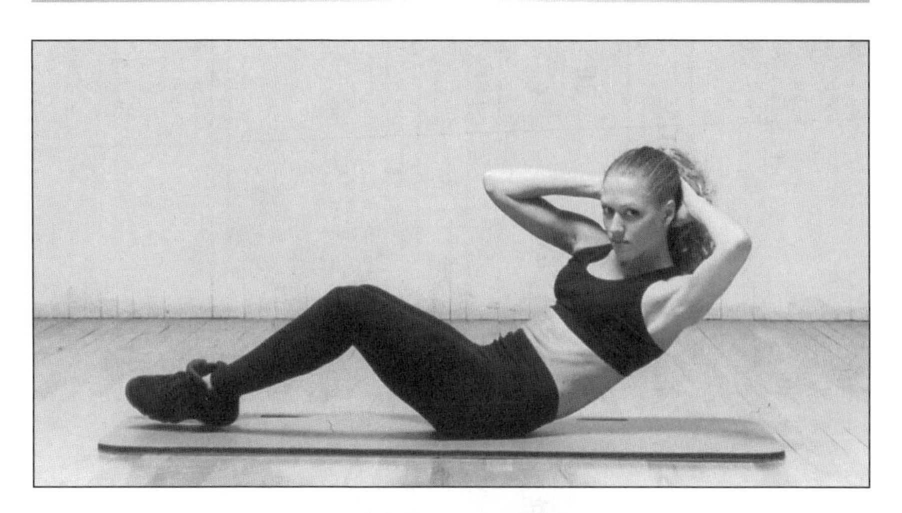

Ab Fitness (Obliques)
Slow

PREPARATION

- Lie on back.
- Place soles of the feet together, as close to the buttocks as possible. The closer the feet are to the buttocks, the more difficult the exercise.
- Drop knees to the sides into the butterfly position.
- Tilt head back, focusing eyes on the ceiling.
- Place hands behind the head.

ACTION

- Lift the shoulder blades off the floor and twist the upper torso and elbow toward the opposite knee.
- Return to the starting position.
- Continue toward the same side for one set.
- Repeat on the opposite side.

Knee-Ups

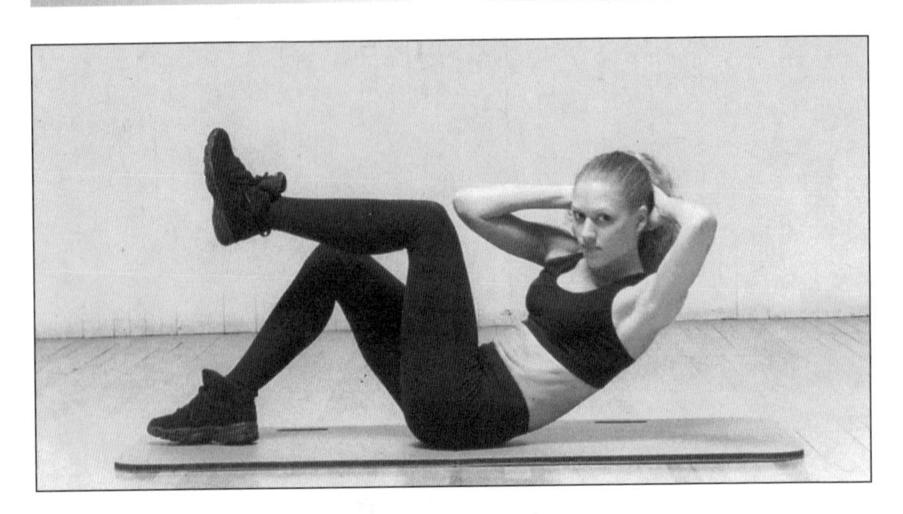

Ab Fitness (Obliques)
Slow to Moderate

PREPARATION

- Lie on back.
- Flex right knee to 90 degrees, placing the right foot flat on the floor.
- Keep left leg straight, approximately six inches off the floor.
- Tuck chin to the chest.
- Place hands behind the head.

ACTION

- Simultaneously lift the upper body and bend the left knee to a midposition and raise the shoulders one to two feet off the floor.
- Twist and tap the right elbow to the left knee.
- Return to the starting position.
- Continue toward the same side for one set.
- Repeat toward the opposite side.

Oblique Leg Roll

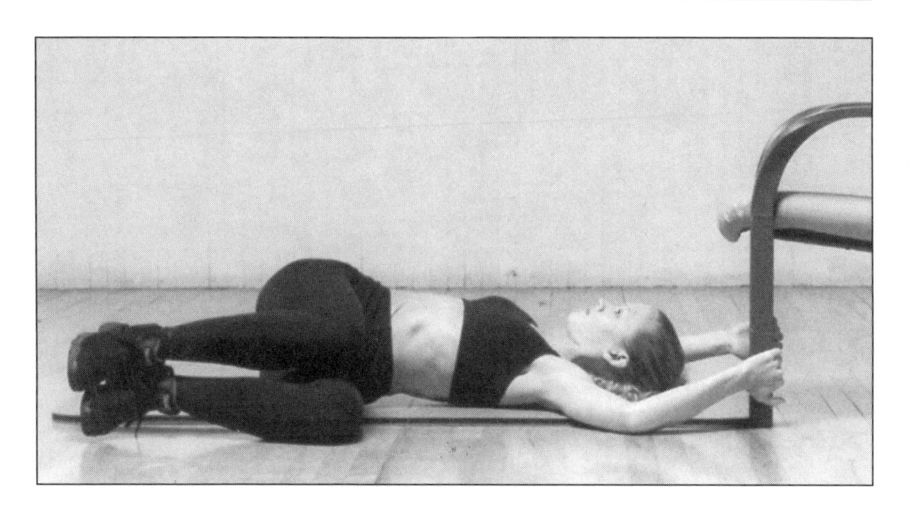

Ab Fitness (Obliques)
Slow

PREPARATION

- Lie on back.
- Tuck both knees toward the chest.
- Place hands either behind the head or extend the arms overhead and hold onto a heavy object, such as a chair, sofa, or bed frame for stability.
- Keep shoulders flat on the floor.

ACTION

- Keeping the knees tucked toward the chest, slowly lower the legs to the left side.
- Touch the floor, then return to the starting position.
- Continue to isolate the left side or alternate sides.

Note: Do not pull with the arms. Keep the shoulders in contact with the floor throughout the set.

Broomstick Twist

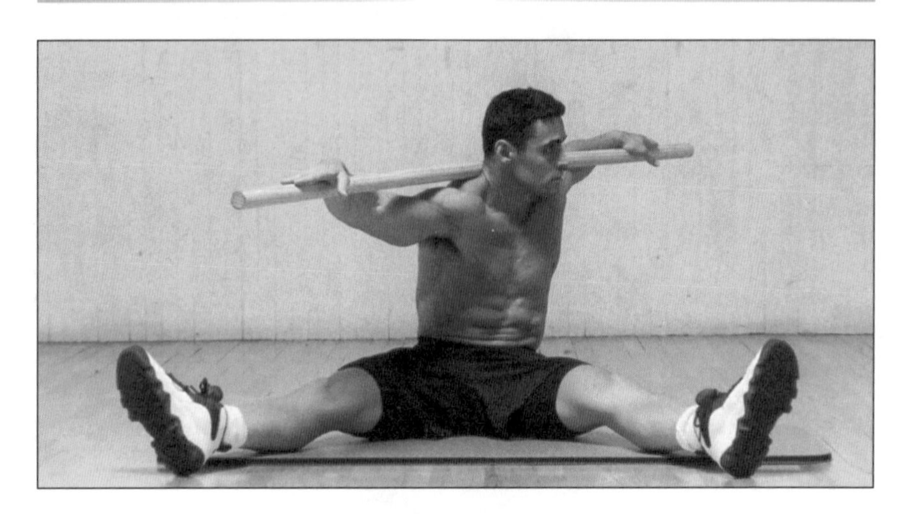

Ab Fitness (Obliques)
Slow

PREPARATION

- Sit tall on the floor.
- Spread legs.
- Hold broomstick across the shoulders.

ACTION

- Contract the obliques and rotate the trunk and torso to the left.
- Return to the starting position.
- Continue to isolate the left side or alternate sides.

Broomstick Oblique Crunch

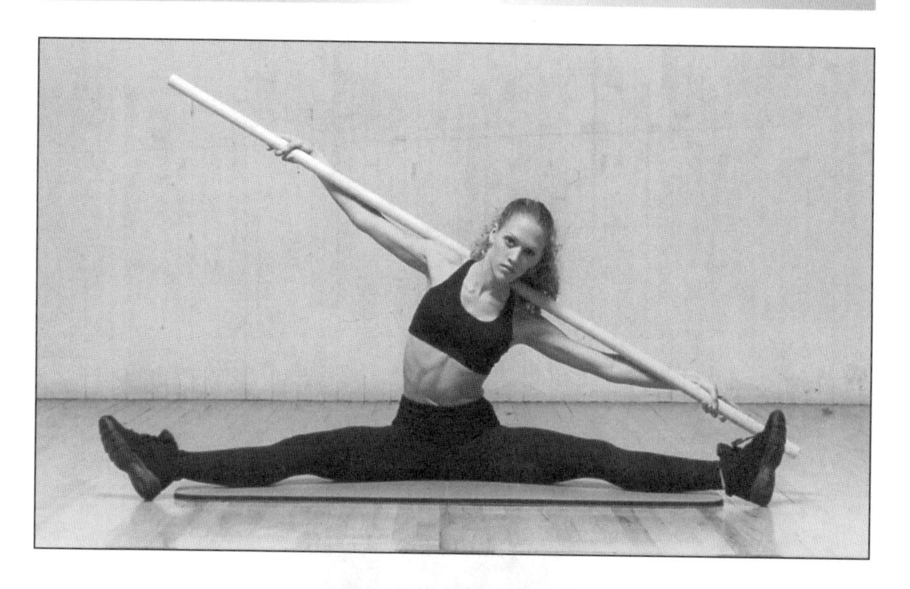

Ab Fitness (Obliques)
Slow

PREPARATION

- Sit tall on the floor.
- Spread legs.
- Hold broomstick across the shoulders.

ACTION

- Contract the left obliques and crunch to the left side.
- Hold for one count.
- Return to the starting position.
- Continue to isolate the left side or alternate sides.

Note: This is a very good *beginning* oblique exercise.

Roll Back Using Momentum

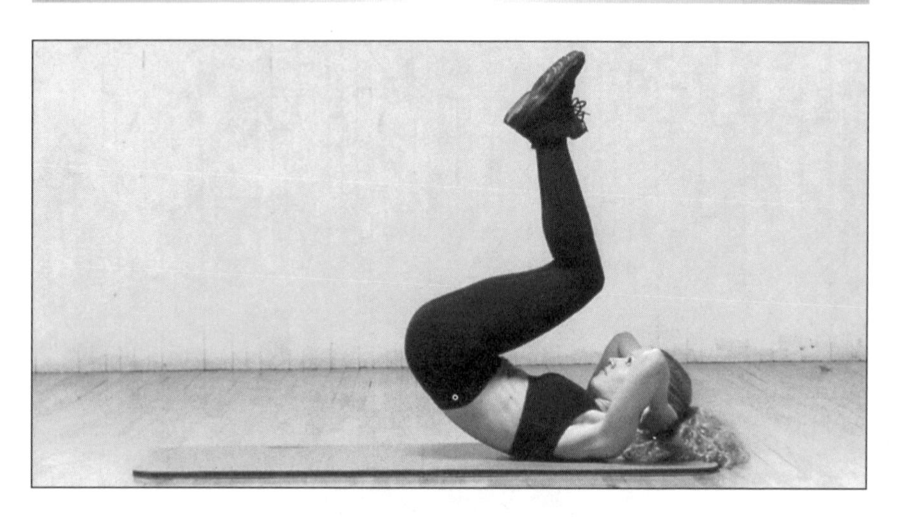

Ab Fitness (Lower)
Slow to Moderate

PREPARATION

- Lie on back.
- Flex knees to 90 degrees.
- Keep feet flat on the floor.
- Tuck chin to the chest.
- Raise shoulders (but not shoulder blades) slightly off the floor.
- Place hands behind the head.

ACTION

- Concentrating on the lower abs, rock the legs back toward the chest, simultaneously lifting (thrusting) the pelvis toward the ceiling.
- Control the contraction, slowly lowering the pelvis and legs back down to the starting position. Keep the spine in contact with the floor.
- Gently tap the feet to the floor and repeat the movement.
- Do not raise the shoulder blades off the floor at any time during the exercise.

Note: As you grow stronger, don't rely on momentum to do this exercise. If you are a beginner, place your hands on the floor under your pelvis to assist with the lift.

Roll Back Isolate

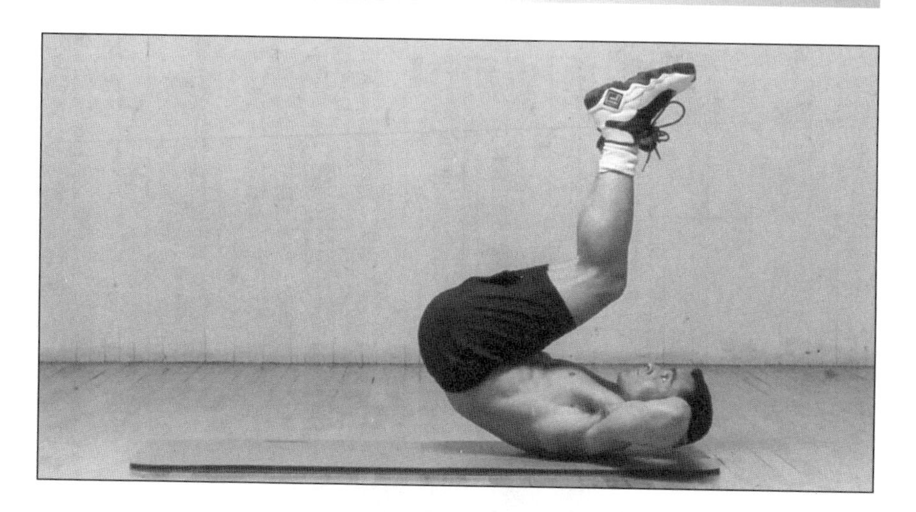

Ab Fitness (Lower)
Slow to Moderate

PREPARATION

- Lie on back.
- Tuck heels close to the buttocks with both feet off the floor.
- Tuck chin to the chest.
- Raise shoulders (but not shoulder blades) off the floor.
- Place hands behind the head.

ACTION

- Isolating the lower abs, pull the legs back toward the shoulders, simultaneously lifting (thrusting) the pelvis toward the ceiling.
- Control the contraction, slowly lowering the pelvis back down to the starting position.
- Don't raise the shoulder blades off the floor at any time during the exercise.

Seated Bent-Knee Tuck

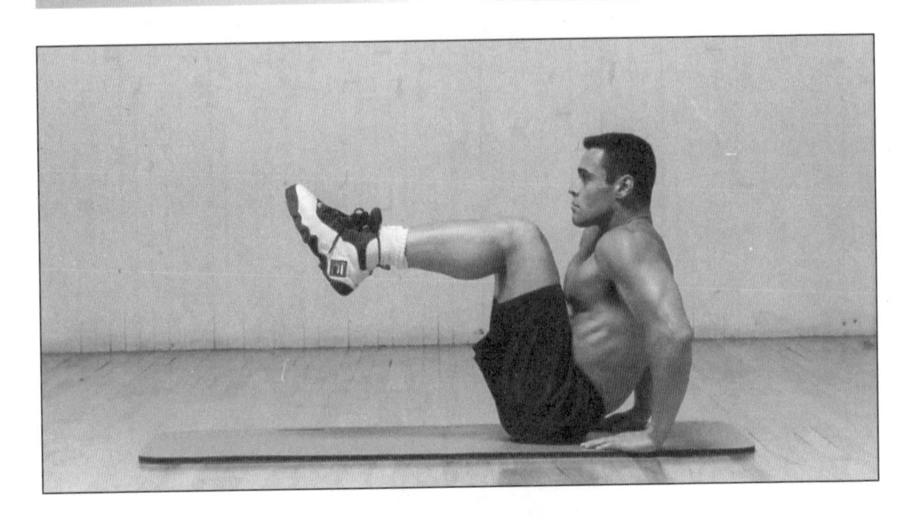

Ab Fitness (Lower)
Slow

PREPARATION

- Sit, leaning back.
- Place the hands on the floor behind the hips to stabilize the upper body.
- Flex knees to 90 degrees.
- Place heels on the floor.

ACTION

- Contract the lower abs and raise the legs to the chest (do not lean further back during the lift).
- Focus on crunching the lower abs. Avoid using the psoas (hip flexor muscles) or momentum to assist with this exercise.
- Do not hyperextend the low back.
- Slowly return to the starting position.
- Immediately repeat.

Note: To make this exercise progressive as you grow stronger, extend the knees more, thus placing a greater workload demand on the lower abs. For example, try flexing the knees to only 100 degrees, then 110, and so on, until you can do this exercise with straight legs.

Seated Straight-Leg Tuck

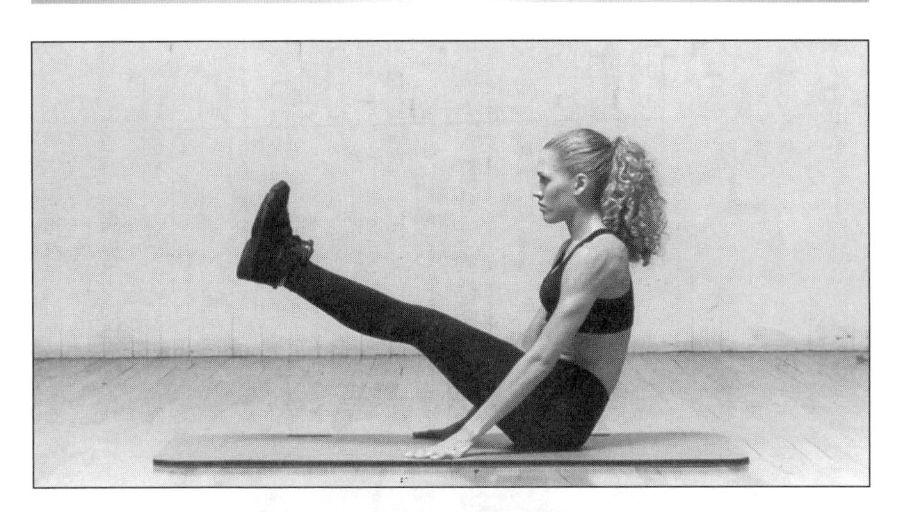

Ab Fitness (Lower)
Slow

PREPARATION

- Unlike the leaning position of the previous Seated Bent-Knee Tuck exercise, this drill requires a more perpendicular posture of the upper body.
- Keep hands on the floor but in *front* of the hips, close to the knees.
- Rest extended legs on the floor.

ACTION

- Contract the lower abs and lift the straight legs as high as possible off the floor.
- Do not hyperextend the low back.
- Hold the up position for one count.
- Slowly lower the legs to the starting position.
- Gently tap the floor.
- Immediately repeat.

Leg Thrusts

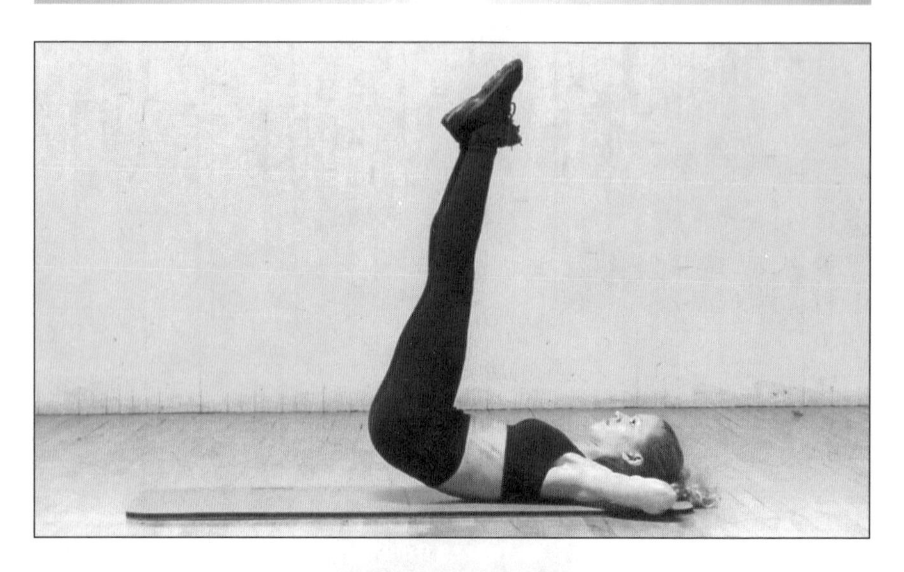

Ab Fitness (Lower)
Slow to Moderate

PREPARATION

- Lie on the floor.
- Flex hips to 90 degrees.
- Extend knees, keeping upper and lower legs perpendicular to the floor.
- Place hands behind the head.

ACTION

- Isolate the lower abs and thrust the legs toward the ceiling.
- Do not rock back onto the shoulders in an effort to assist with the movement.
- Slowly lower the hips to the floor and repeat.

Note: If you need some assistance, extend the arms overhead and hold onto a heavy object, such as a chair, sofa, or bed frame for added leverage.

Cycling

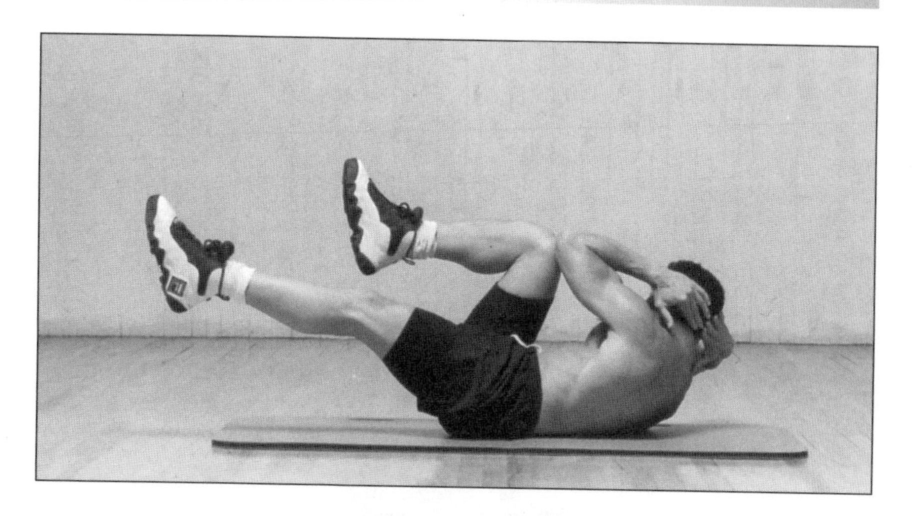

Ab Fitness (Lower)
Moderate to Fast

PREPARATION

- Lie on back.
- Flex hips and knees to 90 degrees.
- Raise shoulder blades several inches off the floor.
- Place hands behind the head.

ACTION

- Extend the left knee while simultaneously driving the right knee in the opposite direction toward the shoulder.
- Tap the right knee with the left elbow.
- Immediately repeat toward the other side.

Note: As you grow stronger, lift the entire back off the floor. Do not exceed a 45-degree angle.

Crossed-Leg Low Ab Crunch

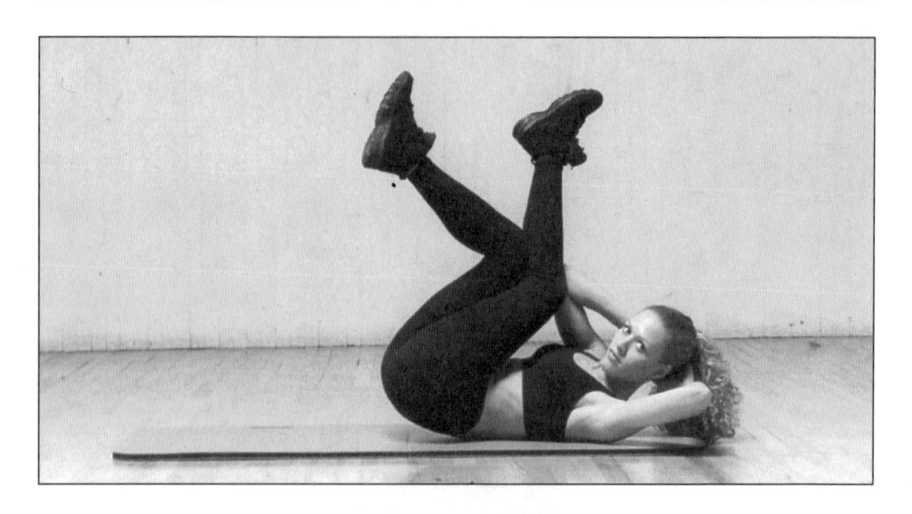

Ab Fitness (Lower)
Slow to Moderate

PREPARATION

- Lie on back.
- Cross the left leg over the right.
- Lift both legs (don't let feet touch the floor).
- Place hands behind the head.

ACTION

- Concentrating on the lower abs, lift the left leg back toward the right shoulder.
- Simultaneously lift the upper body and twist the right elbow toward the left knee.
- Control the contraction, slowly concurrently lowering the pelvis, legs, and shoulders back down to the starting position.
- Do not touch the feet to the floor.
- Continue on the same side until you finish the set.
- Repeat on the opposite side.

Note: As you grow stronger, don't rely on momentum to do this exercise. If you are a beginner, place your hands on the floor under your pelvis to assist with the lift.

Wrist-Ups

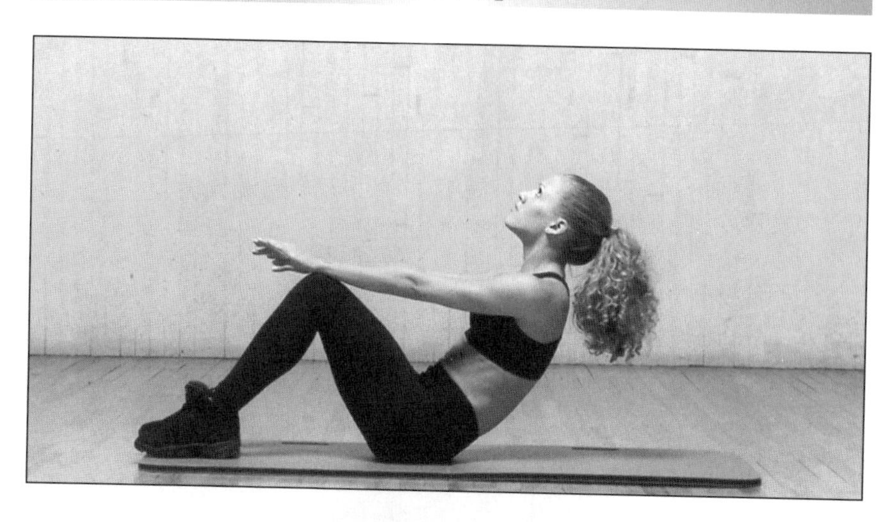

Ab Fitness (Upper)
Slow

PREPARATION

- Lie on back.
- Flex knees to 90 degrees.
- Keep feet flat on the floor.
- Place hands on the thighs.
- Tuck chin to the chest.
- Raise shoulders (not shoulder blades) off the floor.

ACTION

- Slowly (two counts) lift the upper body off the floor, sliding the hands along the thighs until the wrists crest the knees.
- Allow the head to drop back away from the chest when in the up position.
- Hold for one count.
- Slowly (two to four counts) return to the starting position.
- Tap the shoulder blades to the floor (do not bounce).
- Immediately repeat.
- Keep the abs tight at all times.

Ab Curl

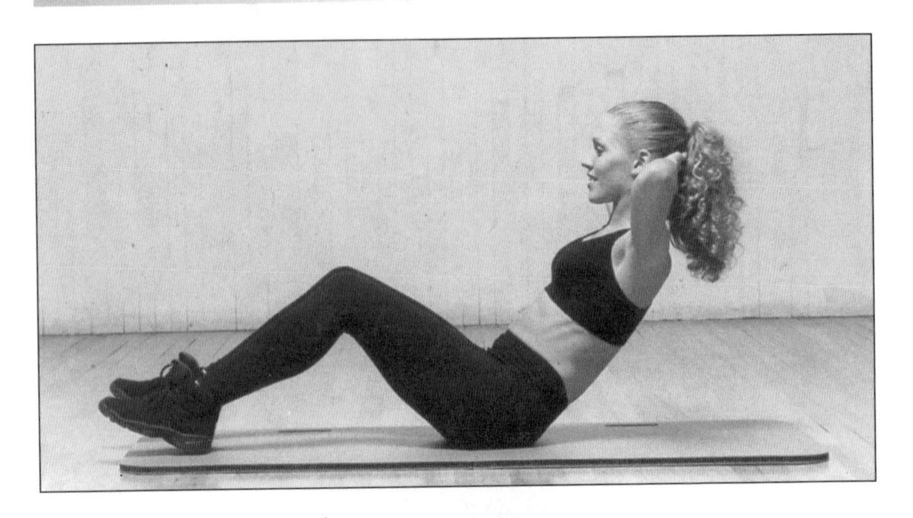

Ab Fitness (Upper)
Slow

PREPARATION

- Flex knees to 90 degrees.
- Place feet flat on the floor.
- Keep head back throughout the exercise.
- Place hands behind the head.

ACTION

- Contract the abs and lift the shoulders and upper body to a position approximately 30 degrees from the floor.
- Hold for one count.
- Return to the starting position.
- Immediately repeat.

Note: Do not pull on the head or neck.

90-Degree Support Crunches

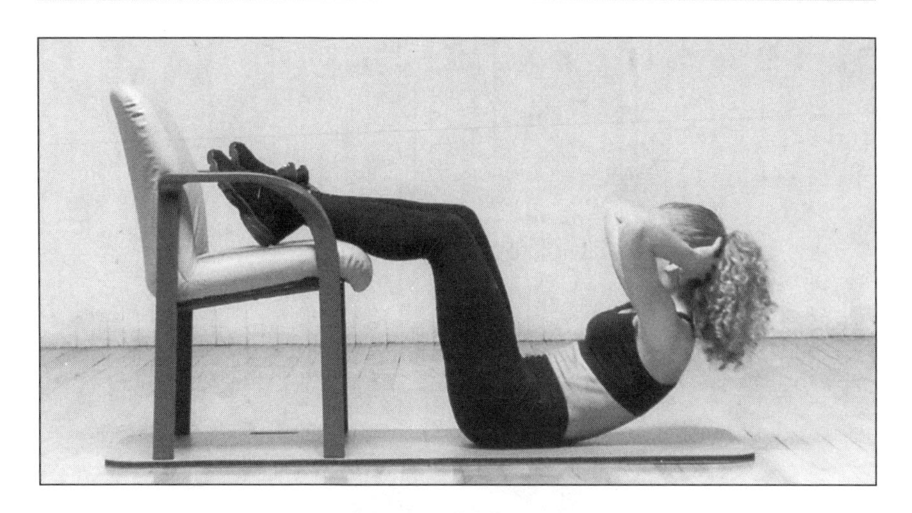

Ab Fitness (Upper)
Slow

PREPARATION

- Lie on back.
- Flex hips and knees to 90 degrees.
- Rest lower legs on a support, such as a chair, bed, sofa, or partner, to provide stability but do not hook the feet.
- Keep buttocks as close as possible to the support.
- Tuck chin to the chest.
- Tilt head back, focusing eyes on the ceiling.
- Place hands behind the head.

ACTION

- Lift the upper body to a position approximately 30 degrees off the floor. (As you grow stronger, tap the elbows to the knees.)
- Slowly return to the starting position.
- Tap the shoulder blades to the floor (do not bounce).
- Immediately repeat.
- Do not pull on the head or neck.

Note: The farther the buttocks are from the support, the less difficult the exercise. As you grow stronger, place the feet against a wall, then eliminate the support altogether. However, always maintain the 90-degree hip and knee flexion.

90-Degree Crunches Without Support

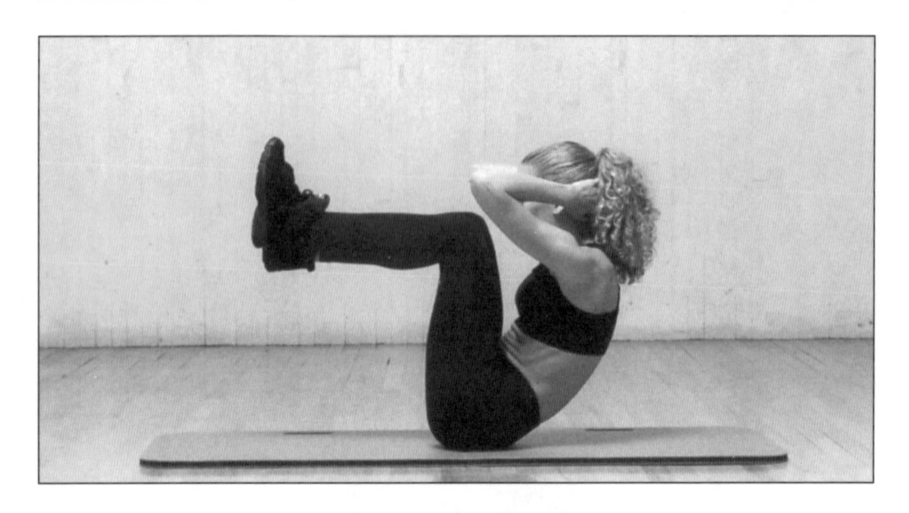

Ab Fitness (Upper)
Slow to Moderate

PREPARATION

- Lie on back.
- Flex hips and knees to 90 degrees.
- Tilt head back, focusing eyes on the ceiling.
- Place hands behind the head.

ACTION

- Lift the upper body to a position approximately 30 degrees off the floor. (As you grow stronger, tap the elbows to the knees.)
- Raise the upper body toward the knees; do not move the knees down toward the upper body.
- Slowly return to the starting position.
- Tap the shoulder blades to the floor (do not bounce).
- Immediately repeat.
- Do not pull on the head or neck.

Butterfly Curl-Up

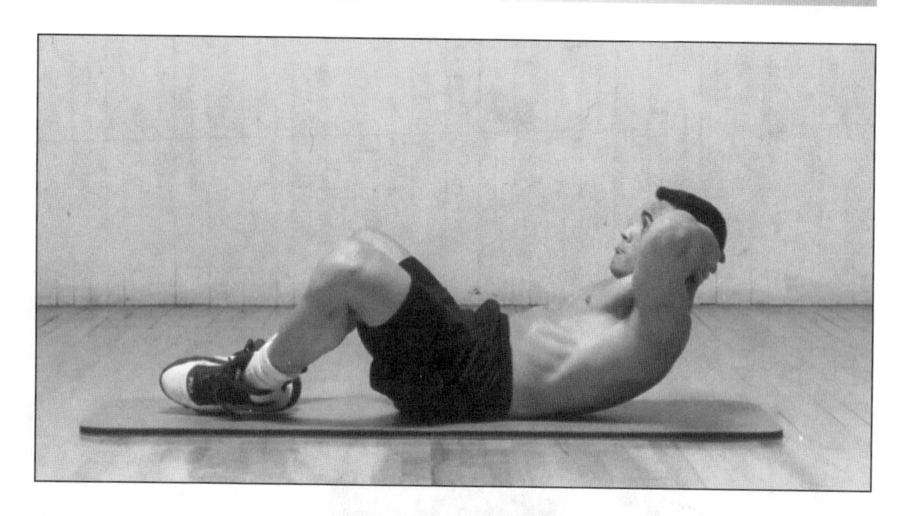

Ab Fitness (Upper)
Slow

PREPARATION

- Lie on back.
- Place soles of the feet together, as close to the buttocks as possible.
- Drop knees to the sides into the butterfly position.
- Tilt head back, focusing eyes on the ceiling.
- Place hands behind the head.

ACTION

- Contract the upper abs and lift the shoulder blades to a position approximately 30 degrees off the floor.
- Return to the starting position.
- Tap the shoulder blades to the floor (do not bounce).
- Immediately repeat.

Note: Remember, experiment with different arm positions to vary the difficulty of this and all other exercises. Start with the arms extended, reaching between the legs. As you grow stronger, fold the arms across the chest, then advance to putting them behind the head. You can manipulate the positions of the legs and feet (extended or up close to the buttocks) to create greater leverage, thereby assisting in the movement. Hooking the feet can be of great help to the beginner.

135-Degree Wall Reach

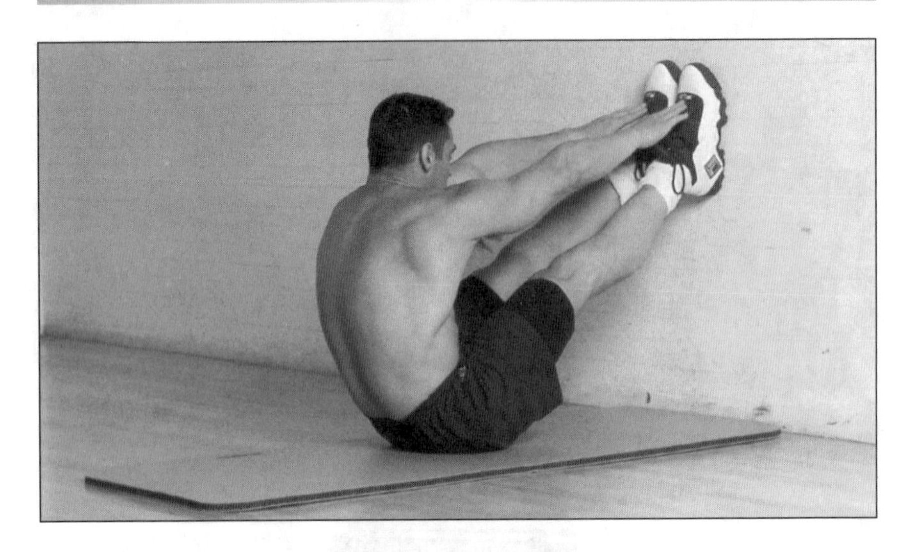

Ab Fitness (Upper)
Slow to Moderate

PREPARATION

- Lie on back.
- Rest feet lightly on wall with legs straight.
- Keep hip angle at approximately 135 degrees.
- Extend arms toward the feet.
- Keep hands together.
- Focus eyes on the feet.

ACTION

- Crunch the upper abs by raising the upper body and reaching toward the feet.
- Tap the feet.
- Slowly return to the starting position.
- Immediately repeat.

Note: This exercise is typically performed with the arms extended as outlined but you may position the hands across the chest or behind the head to increase the resistance.

90-Degree Wall Reach

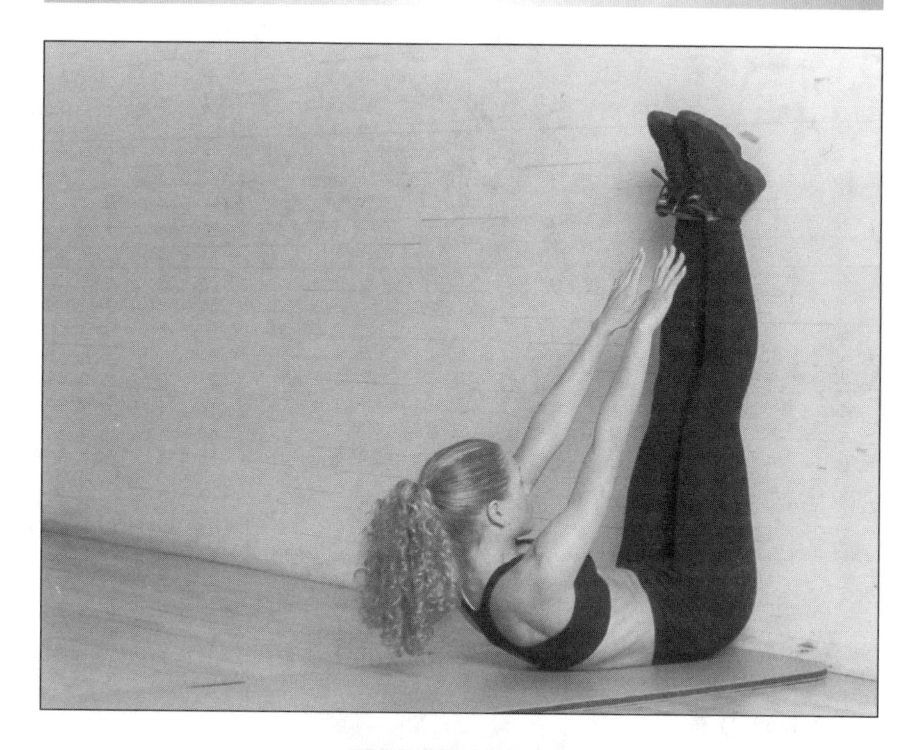

Ab Fitness (Upper)
Moderate

PREPARATION

- Keep legs straight.
- Keep hip angle at 90 degrees, with legs perpendicular to the floor.
- Slide as close to the wall as possible, touching buttocks to the wall.
- Extend arms toward the feet.
- Keep hands together.
- Focus eyes on the feet.

ACTION

- Crunch the upper abs and raise the upper body, reaching toward the feet.
- Tap the feet.
- Return to the starting position.
- Immediately repeat.

Note: This exercise is typically performed with the arms extended as outlined but you may position the hands across the chest or behind the head to increase the resistance.

Toes to Ceiling

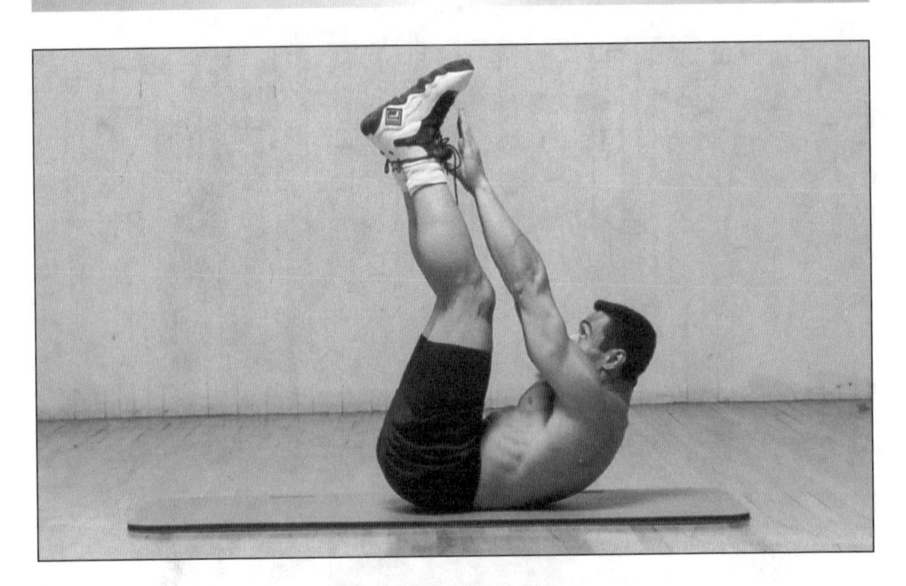

Ab Fitness (Upper)
Slow to Moderate

PREPARATION

- Lie on back.
- Keep legs straight.
- Keep hip angle at 90 degrees, with legs perpendicular to the floor.
- Extend arms toward the feet.
- Keep hands together.
- Focus eyes on the feet.

ACTION

- Crunch the upper abs and raise the upper body, reaching toward the feet.
- Tap the feet and return to the starting position.
- Immediately repeat.
- To incorporate the obliques, reach across toward the opposite foot.

Note: This exercise is typically performed with the arms extended as outlined but you may position the hands across the chest or behind the head to increase the resistance.

Single-Leg Bent-Knee Jackknives

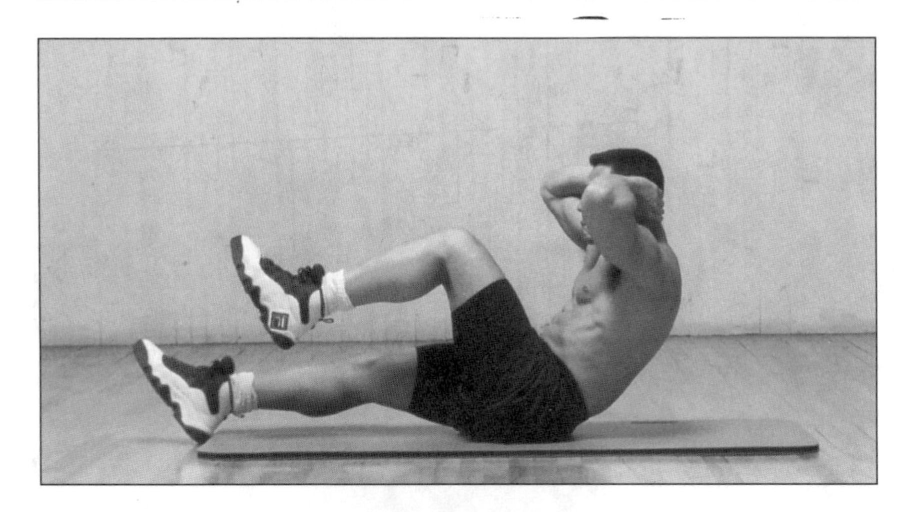

Ab Fitness (Upper)
Slow to Moderate

PREPARATION

- Lie on back.
- Keep both legs straight, heels touching the floor.
- Tuck chin to the chest.
- Raise shoulders off the floor (this will help alleviate hyperextension of the low back).
- Place hands behind the head.

ACTION

- Simultaneously lift the upper body and bend the left knee to a jackknife, or midposition, raising the shoulders one to two feet off the floor.
- Tap the left elbow with the left knee.
- Return to the starting position. (Keep the shoulders off the floor; do not hyperextend the low back.)
- Continue on the same side for one set.
- Repeat on the opposite side.

Note: If you feel too much stress in the low back, try flexing the right knee to 90 degrees and keeping the right foot flat on the floor throughout the exercise.

Double-Leg Bent-Knee Jackknives

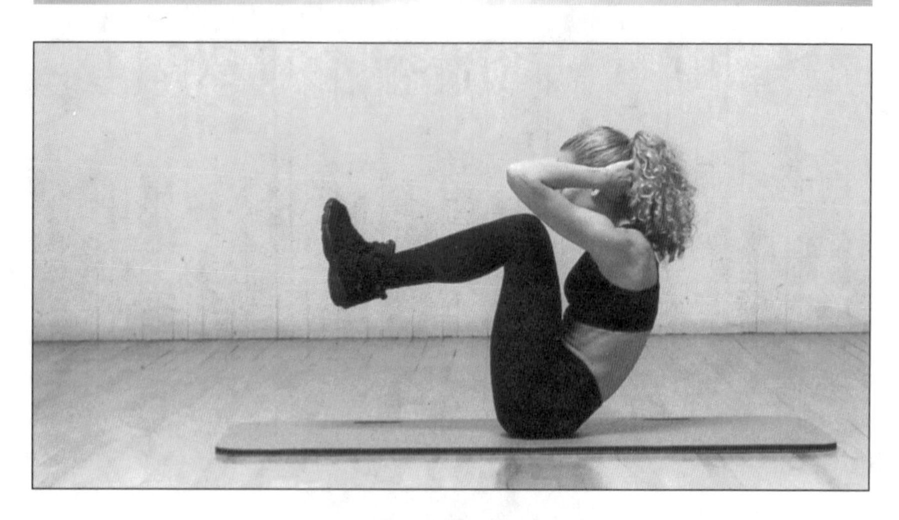

Ab Fitness (Upper)
Slow to Moderate

PREPARATION

- Lie on back.
- Keep both legs straight, heels touching the floor.
- Tuck chin to the chest.
- Raise shoulders off the floor (this will help alleviate hyperextension of the low back).
- Place hands behind the head.

ACTION

- Simultaneously lift the upper body and bend both legs to a midposition, raising the shoulders one to two feet off the floor.
- Touch the elbows to the knees.
- Return to the starting position. (Keep the shoulder blades off the floor; do not hyperextend the low back.)
- Immediately repeat.

Note: Avoid this exercise if you experience any low back stress.

Single-Leg Straight-Leg Jackknives

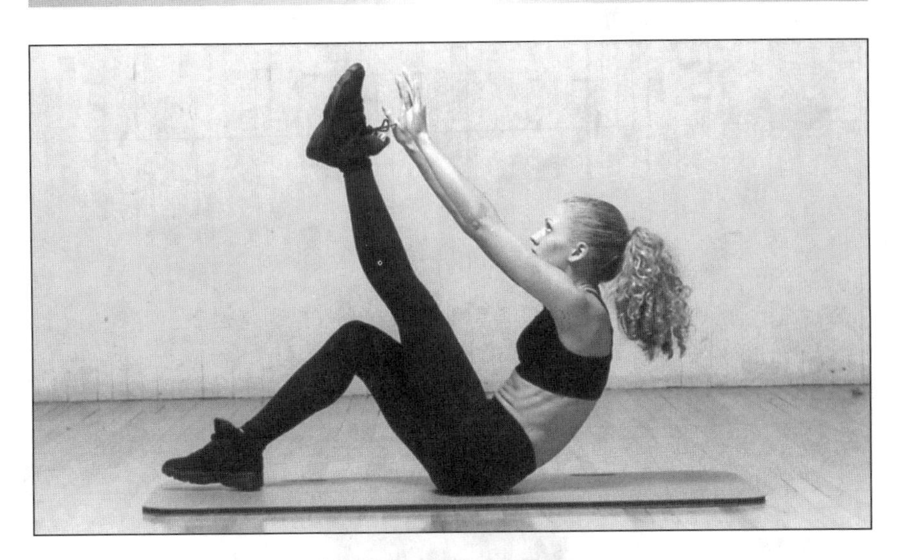

Ab Fitness (Upper)
Slow to Moderate

PREPARATION

- Lie on back.
- Flex right knee to 90 degrees, keeping the right foot flat on the floor.
- Keep left leg straight with left heel touching the floor.
- Extend arms overhead.

ACTION

- Simultaneously lift the upper body and the straight left leg to midposition, raising the shoulders one to two feet off the floor.
- Touch hands to the left foot.
- Return to the starting position.
- Continue on the same side for one set.
- Repeat on the opposite side.

Note: Avoid "throwing" the arms; rather, isolate the abs and lift the upper body to the correct position.

Russian Twist

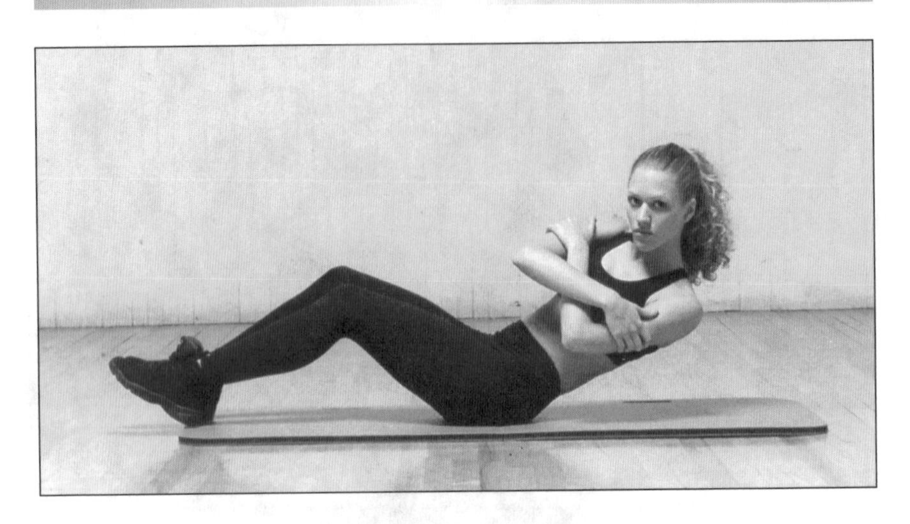

Ab Fitness (Upper)
Slow

PREPARATION

- Lie on back.
- Flex knees to between 90 and 120 degrees.
- Place feet flat on the floor.
- Fold arms across the chest.
- Begin the movement with the upper body approximately 30 degrees off the floor.

ACTION

- Twist the upper body to the left.
- Raise the upper body from the 30-degree position to approximately 45 degrees off the floor.
- Hold this position for one count.
- Twist to the right.
- Lower the upper body from 45 to 30 degrees.
- Hold this position for one count.
- Twist to the left.
- Continue same rotation until all repetitions in the set have been completed.
- Repeat to the opposite rotation.

Negatives

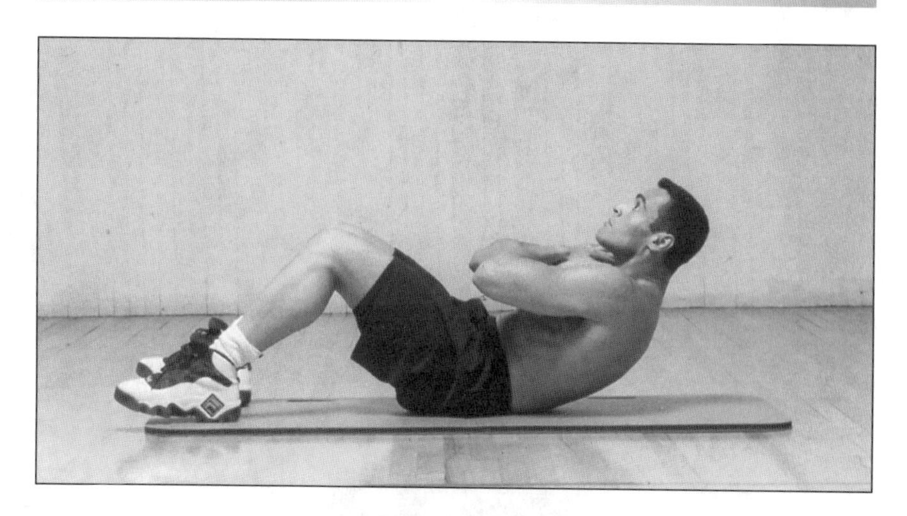

Ab Fitness (Upper)
Slow

PREPARATION

- Flex knees to 90 degrees.
- Place feet flat on the floor.
- Fold arms across the chest.
- Begin the movement with the upper body approximately 45 degrees off the floor.

ACTION

- *Slowly* (count five) lower the upper body to the floor.
- Tap the shoulder blades (do not bounce).
- Quickly return to the starting position.
- Immediately repeat.

Note: Beginners may need to hook their feet until adequate strength levels are developed. As fatigue sets in, avoid hyperextending the low back.

Low Back Isolate

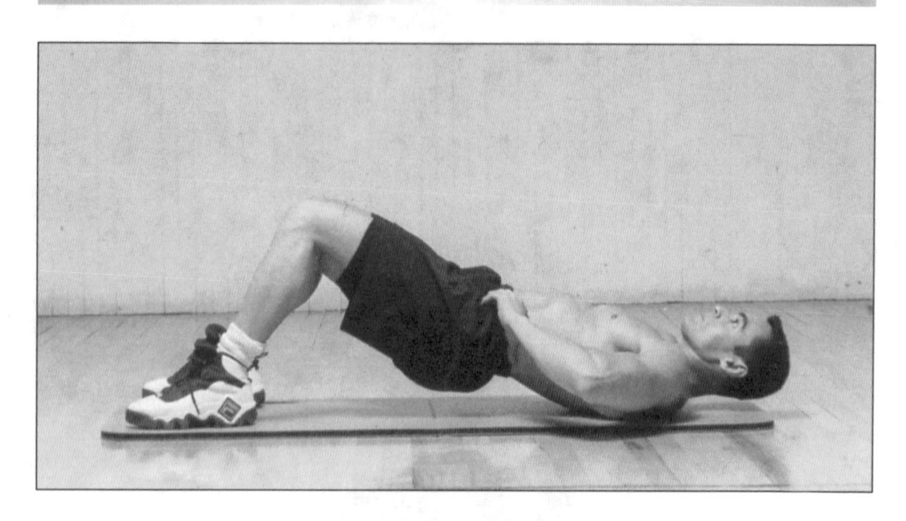

Ab Fitness (Back)
Slow

PREPARATION

- Lie on the floor in a supine position with entire spine in contact with the floor.
- Flex knees to 90 degrees.
- Place feet flat on the floor, shoulder-width apart.
- Place hands on the hips.

ACTION

- Contract the low back muscles and gluteals and lift the hips off the floor.
- Keep the shoulders and upper back in contact with the floor.
- Keep body weight off the neck.
- Hold for 5 to 10 counts.
- Return to the starting position.
- Immediately repeat.

Note: Place a pillow under the head and neck for added comfort and support.

Low Back Isolate: Contract-Relax

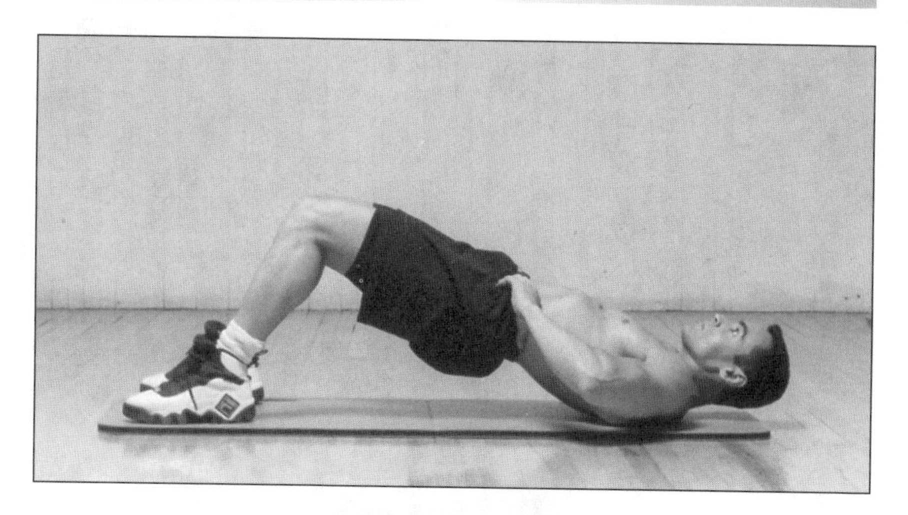

Ab Fitness (Back)
Slow

PREPARATION

- Lie on back.
- Flex knees to 90 degrees.
- Place feet on the floor, shoulder-width apart.
- Place hands on the hips.

ACTION

- Contract the low back muscles and gluteals and lift the hips off the floor (see photo on page 126).
- Keep the shoulders and upper back in contact with the floor.
- Keep body weight off the neck.
- From the up position, contract and raise the hips another six to eight inches.
- Hold for one count.
- Return to the up position.
- Immediately repeat.

Note: Place a pillow under the head and neck for added comfort and support.

Prone Leg Lift

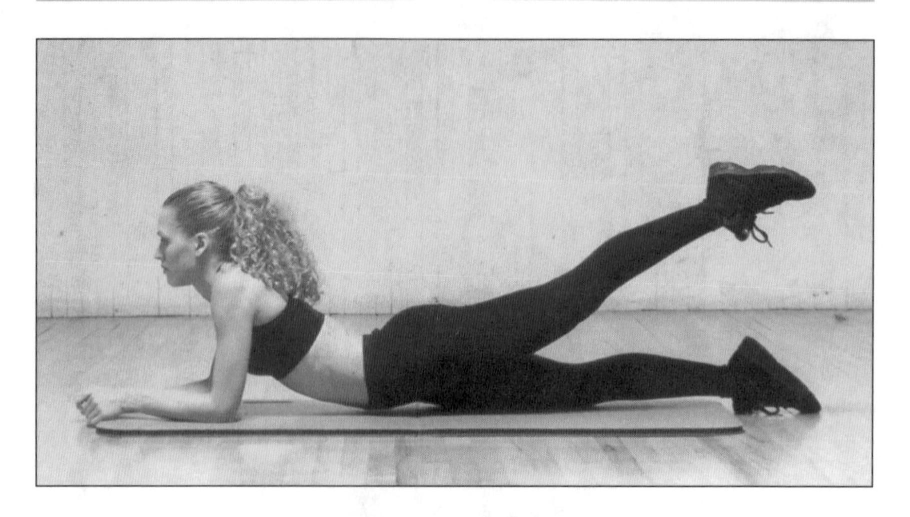

Ab Fitness (Back)
Slow

PREPARATION

- Lie on the floor in a prone position.
- Lightly support the upper body with the elbows.

ACTION

- Contract the left gluteal and hamstring and lift the straight leg as high as comfortably possible.
- Hold for one count.
- Return to the starting position.
- Either continue on the same side for one set or alternate sides.

Back Crunch

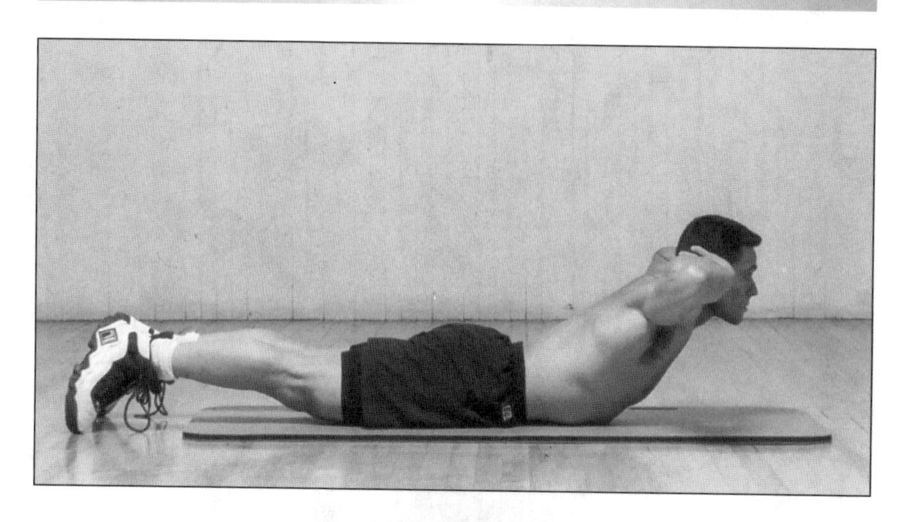

Ab Fitness (Back)
Slow

PREPARATION

- Lie on the floor in a prone position.
- Place hands behind the head.

ACTION

- Contract the low back muscles and gluteals.
- Lift the upper body so that the chest is three to four inches off the floor.
- Hold for one count.
- Slowly return to the starting position.
- Immediately repeat.

Note: Beginners having difficulty performing this exercise because of low strength levels might try hooking the feet or having a partner apply light pressure to the ankles for added leverage. If you are still having trouble, try positioning the arms at the sides before advancing on to the more difficult "hands behind the head" position.

Back Crunch Twist

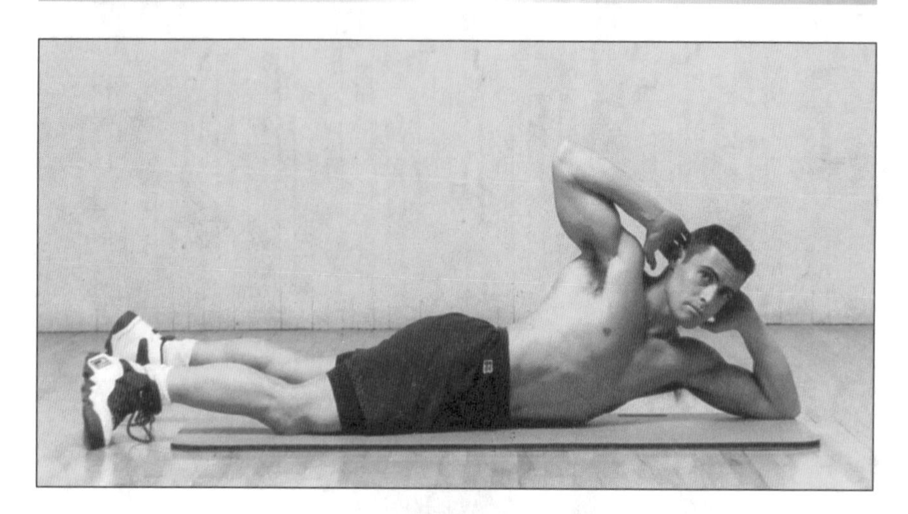

Ab Fitness (Back)
Slow

PREPARATION

- Lie on the floor in a prone position.
- Spread legs, feet shoulder-width apart.
- Place hands behind the head, with elbows touching the floor.

ACTION

- Isolate the left gluteal and low back muscles.
- Keep the left elbow in contact with the floor.
- Lift and twist.
- Hold for one count.
- Slowly return to the starting position.
- Either continue toward the same side for one set or alternate sides.
- As strength levels improve, keep both elbows off the floor during the movement.

Note: Beginners having difficulty performing this exercise because of low strength levels might try hooking the feet or having a partner apply light pressure to the ankles for added leverage.

Superman

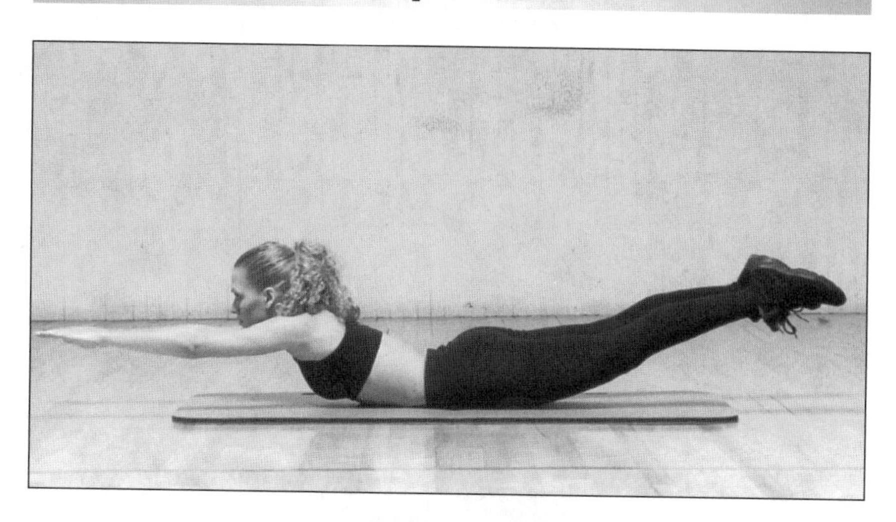

Ab Fitness (Back)
Slow

PREPARATION

- Lie on the floor in a prone position.
- Extend arms overhead.

ACTION

- Simultaneously lift the upper body and the legs off the floor.
- Hold the contracted position for three to five counts.
- Return to the starting position.
- Immediately repeat.

Unilateral Superman

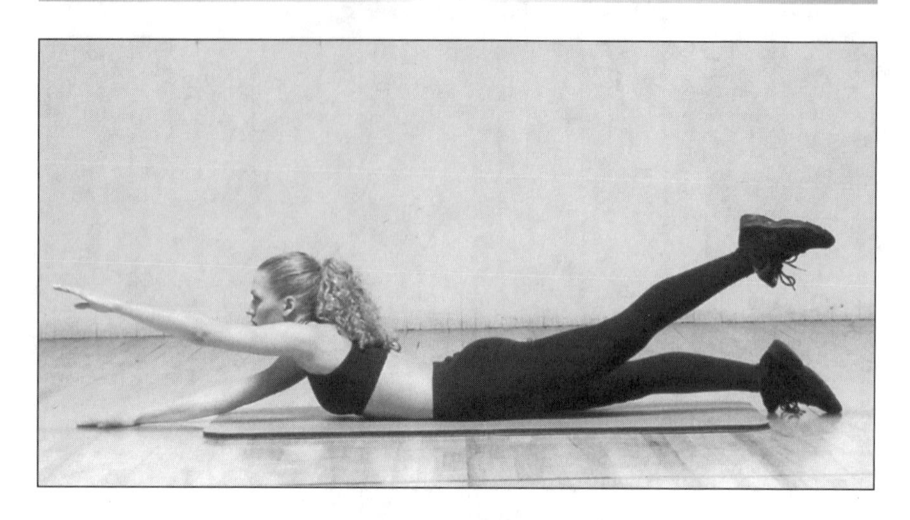

Ab Fitness (Back)
Slow

PREPARATION

- Lie on the floor in a prone position.
- Extend arms overhead.

ACTION

- Simultaneously lift the left arm and upper body and left leg off the floor.
- Hold the contracted position for three to five counts.
- Return to the starting position.
- Either continue on the same side for one set or alternate sides.

Contralateral Superman

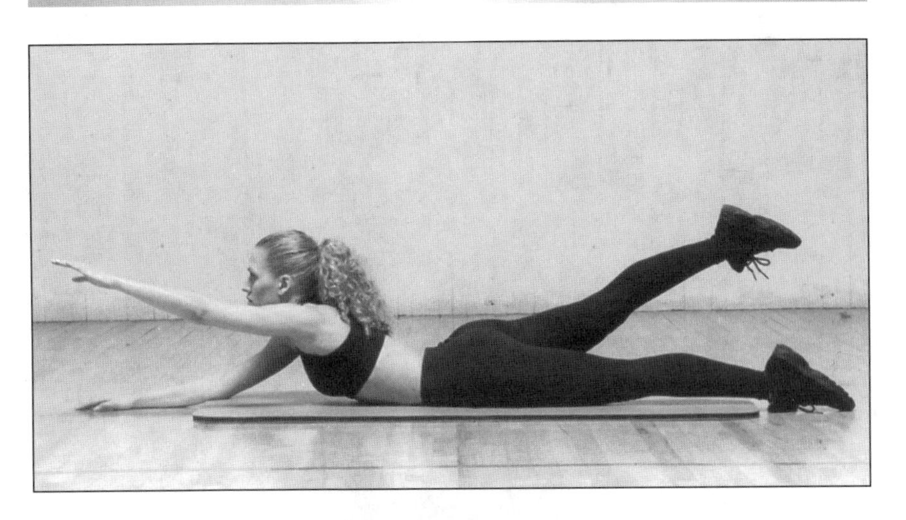

Ab Fitness (Back)
Slow

PREPARATION

- Lie on the floor in a prone position.
- Extend arms overhead.

ACTION

- Simultaneously lift the left arm and upper body and the right leg off the floor.
- Hold the contracted position for three to five counts.
- Return to the starting position.
- Repeat the movement with the opposite extremities (e.g., right arm, left leg).

Side Leg Raise

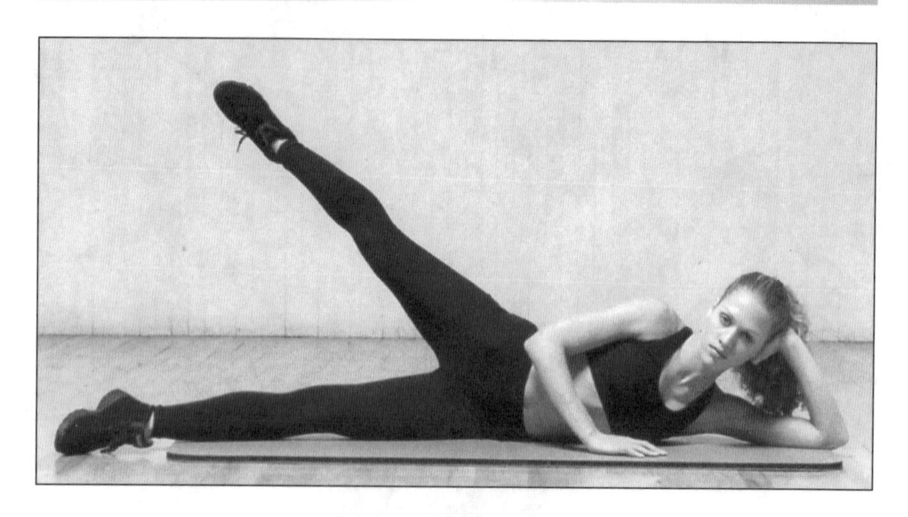

Ab Fitness (Back)
Slow

PREPARATION

- Lie on the left side.
- Keep legs straight.
- Rest left elbow on the floor and the head in the left hand.
- Tilt the body slightly forward.
- Hold right leg approximately 12 inches above the left leg.

ACTION

- Contract the right gluteal and low back muscles and lift the right leg up and back as far as comfortably possible.
- Hold for one count.
- Return to the starting position (right leg 12 inches above the left).
- Continue on the same side for one set.
- Repeat on the opposite side.

Hip Extension

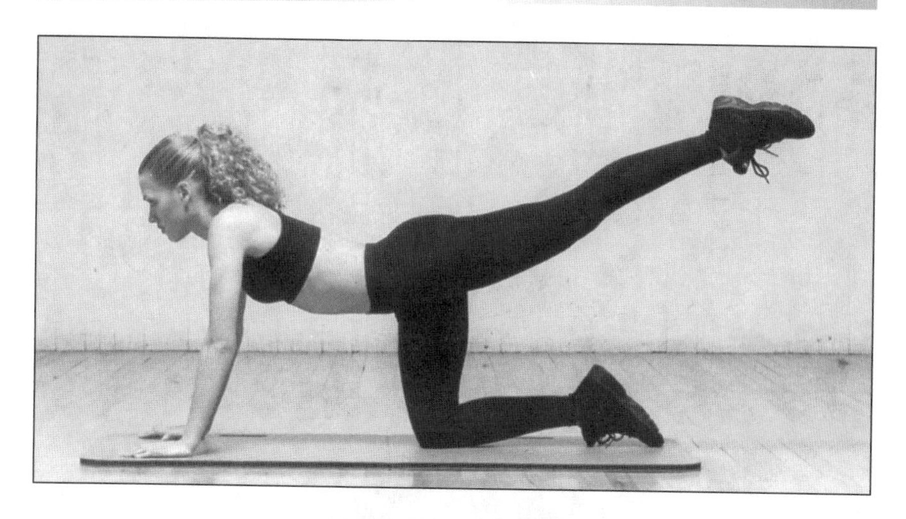

Ab Fitness (Back)
Slow

PREPARATION

- Place hands and right knee on the floor.
- Extend the left leg, with left toes touching the floor.
- Lift head slightly up, focusing eyes about three to four feet ahead on the floor.

ACTION

- Contract the left gluteal and hamstring and lift the leg as high as comfortably possible.
- Hold for one count.
- Return to the starting position.
- Continue on the same side for one set.
- Repeat on the opposite side.

Note: You can perform this exercise from a standing position. Place the hands against a wall and follow the *action* directions listed.

Hip Extension With Knee Tuck

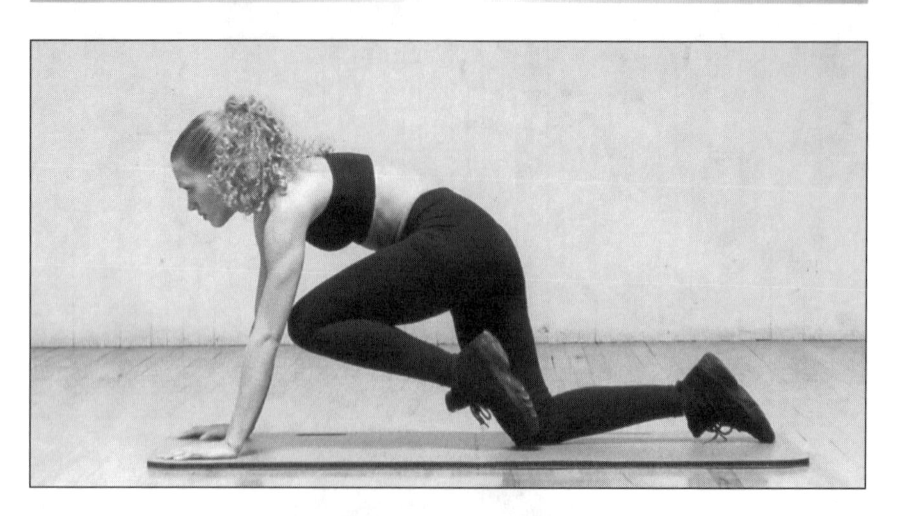

Ab Fitness (Back)
Slow

PREPARATION

- Place hands and right knee on the floor.
- Tuck left leg up under the chest.
- Lift head slightly up, focusing eyes about three to four feet ahead on the floor.

ACTION

- Simultaneously extend and lift the left leg as high as comfortably possible (see photo on page 135).
- Hold for one count.
- Return to the starting position.
- Continue on the same side for one set.
- Repeat on the opposite side.

Note: You can perform this exercise from a standing position. Place the hands against a wall and follow the *action* directions listed.

Partner-Assisted Hyperextension

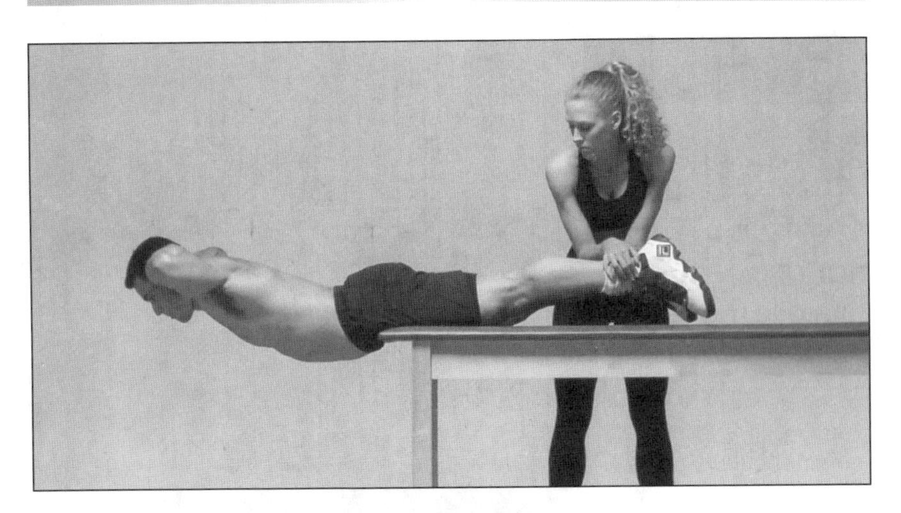

Ab Fitness (Back)
Slow

PREPARATION

- Lie across a firm bed (or padded table) with the legs on the bed and the upper body hanging toward the floor.
- Position the hips at the edge of the bed.
- Have a partner apply pressure to the lower legs.
- Place hands either behind the head or protecting the face. Beginners should use the arms (hands on the floor) to assist with the movement. As strength levels improve, you'll require less assistance until, ultimately, you won't need to use your arms for support.

ACTION

- Contract the low back muscles and gluteals and lift the upper body to a horizontal position.
- Pause for one count with the upper body *parallel* to the floor.
- Slowly return to the starting position.
- Immediately repeat.
- Keep the head and shoulders tilted back throughout the lift.

Bent-Knee Dead Lift

Ab Fitness (Back)
Slow

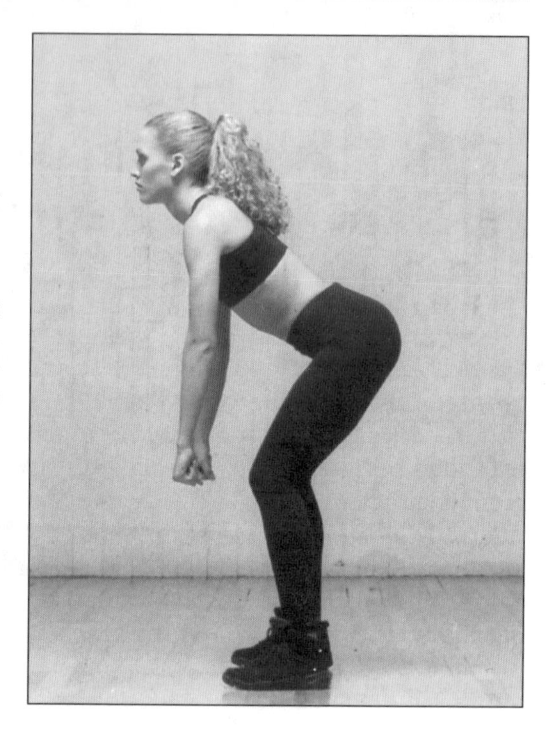

PREPARATION

- Stand erect, feet shoulder-width apart.

ACTION

- With the back straight, flex the hips and bend knees until the hands are positioned slightly below the knees.
- Keep head up.
- Using the legs and low back, stand erect.
- Immediately repeat.

Note: For added resistance try holding a plastic water jug (containing varying amounts of water as dictated by current strength levels) in each hand.

7 Ab Strength Exercises

If you'll recall, absolute muscular strength is the maximum amount of force that a muscle generates in one contraction; and muscular endurance is the ability of muscle to exert force repeatedly over an extended period of time. The degree of muscular strength development is directly related to the degree of the overload. In chapter 1 we referred to the Greek wrestler, Milo of Crotona, and his elementary system of developing strength. As the young calf gradually grew into a bull, Milo had to progressively adapt to the increased resistance as he carried the animal across the arena every day. This is progressive overload. According to this principle, to improve strength, you must apply force against a resistance that is greater than that normally experienced in daily activity or sport performance. Once you have adapted to a certain level of resistance, you must increase the load again to ensure continued progress.

Both increasing the size of skeletal muscle and improving the neural control of the muscular system result in increases in the strength and performance of that muscle. A direct relationship between strength training and increase in the size of muscles exists. This increase is referred to as *hypertrophy*. Men, with their naturally higher levels of testosterone, are more likely to experience hypertrophy through strength training than are women and prepubescent children. Women and children, however, can still achieve significant strength, toning, and power gains through an increase in *muscle involvement* and *motor skill development*. Certainly, whatever the mix of hypertrophy and increased motor skill, these exercise-induced changes enable the muscles to handle stress more efficiently with less chance of injury. Such is the case with the center of power.

Since no training program can develop every aspect of the muscle system equally, you must choose what works for you. A regimen emphasizing high resistance and low repetitions (3 to 6) favors muscular strength development. This routine typically employs a long rest interval between sets to allow for a more complete recovery. Hypertrophy, or training for increased muscular mass, is not that far removed from a strength-oriented routine. To create a hypertrophy training program, select a resistance to accommodate a few more repetitions per set (8 to 12) and take a shorter rest interval between multiple sets. In contrast, a routine of lower resistance and higher repetitions (greater than 10) favors muscle toning and endurance. So what direction should *you* pursue? Consider that the trunk and low torso is a region of the body that benefits greatly from maximal strength, yet the muscles are in continuous use, maintaining balance and stability and supporting the spine, requiring muscular endurance. Because of this everyday, continuous use, we recommend a routine that leans more toward the development of muscular endurance for the general population and many athletes.

If you are a serious athlete, you should usually engage in a combination routine, placing greater emphasis on the strength and power end of the continuum. Given the explosive nature of most sport movements, we recommend that you stress power development of your core. Heavy resistance and ballistic type activities tend to recruit the more explosive fast-twitch fibers, so we recommend that you incorporate more of these kinds of activities into your routine than in one for the fitness enthusiast. (We will discuss power training more thoroughly in chapter 8.)

This chapter is entitled "Ab Strength Exercises" for good reasons. With these drills, we'll place greater emphasis on developing strength and applying that strength to athletics. If, however, you are an advanced fitness enthusiast and are so inclined, you may want to include some of these exercises in your own regimen—but only after you have mastered the exercises in chapter 6. The drills in this chapter will involve the use of strength training equipment such as free weights (e.g., barbells and dumbbells) and other means of variable resistance, such as machinery.

Athletes often prefer free weights because using free weights involves secondary muscles, which help control or stabilize the primary movers during the lift. However, some risk in this type of exercise exists and we suggest free weights only for those who have experience with such methods; we do not recommend free weights for the beginner. A certified trainer can provide proper instruction if you feel uncomfortable with free weight technique.

Through the use of levers or cams, variable resistance machines attempt to match the strength curves of the lifter. Distinct strong and weak points exist throughout the range of motion of a particular muscle and its joint or joints. Theoretically, this type of equipment provides less resistance at joint angles where you are the weakest and greater resistance at points where you are the strongest. These machines are safer than free weights and therefore very popular among fitness enthusiasts. Some of the exercises in this chapter will involve the use of variable resistance machinery. Because of the many movements that the core is capable of performing, and because it would be impossible to pinpoint with any degree of precision an average person's force curve, it is difficult to design machines to exercise the core exclusively. Although the engineers designed the levers or cams with different muscle groups in mind, we can adapt pieces of equipment (non-core) to safely challenge the movements of the core region.

If you don't have access to this equipment, you can do several of the exercises in this chapter just as effectively with rubber bands (Therabands or surgical tubing). This type of training is ideal for the frequent traveler who does not want to miss a workout but lacks an adequate or familiar facility. (See photos below and on page 142.)

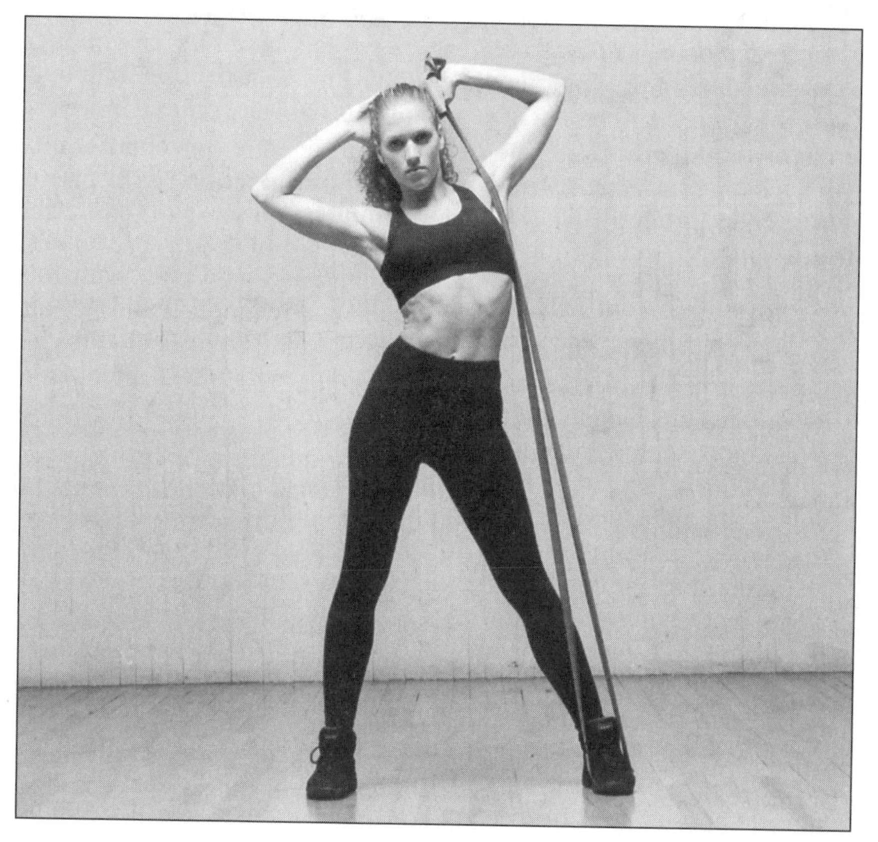

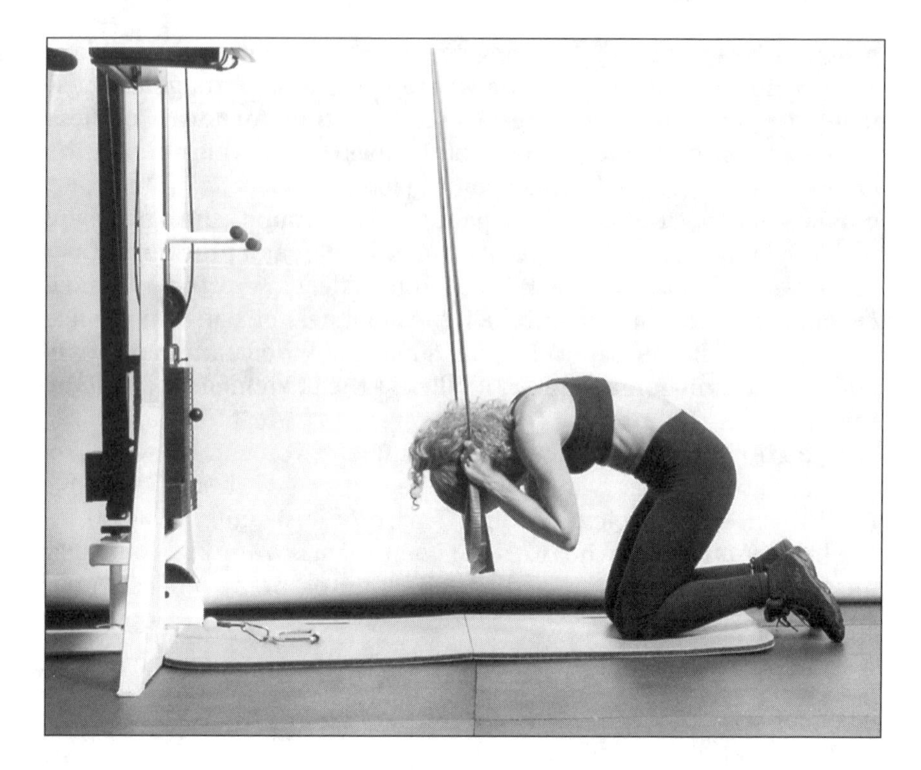

Before you incorporate the exercises outlined in this chapter into your existing program, please review the introduction to chapter 6. Then, keep in mind that we have geared the ab strength exercises toward

- those fitness enthusiasts who are more advanced than most,
- active weekend warriors (those already in good shape), and
- all athletes.

Many of the exercises use external resistance to increase the physical demands on your system. But keep in mind that external resistance also increases the risk of injury. You must take the responsibility for determining if you are capable of executing these exercises safely. Thoroughly review the drill descriptions. If possible, work with an instructor or training partner who is familiar with the correct technique. Practice the movement without the use of external resistance first to ensure that you have the movement down. Work in front of a mirror, instructor, or training partner to get visual or verbal feedback. Once you are comfortable with the technique, slowly incorporate external resistance. Remember: Start with light weights and *never* sacrifice technique for added resistance, repetitions, or sets.

We do not advocate increasing the resistance demands you place on your abdominals and low back to a point that limits you to performing only a few lifts. Increase resistance gradually enough to stress the system progressively while still adhering to the high repetition philosophy.

As with any other type of training, once you stop the program you will experience a rapid detraining effect. You must, at the very least, implement a maintenance program to retain all that you have gained. Fortunately, it's easier to maintain than gain strength. A maintenance program will simply decrease in frequency and duration, but the intensity of the few remaining workouts must stay high. Don't do all the hard work only to turn back into a couch potato. Establish a productive routine and stick with it.

Ab Strength Exercises

Flat Bench Oblique Crunch

Ab Strength (Obliques)
Moderate

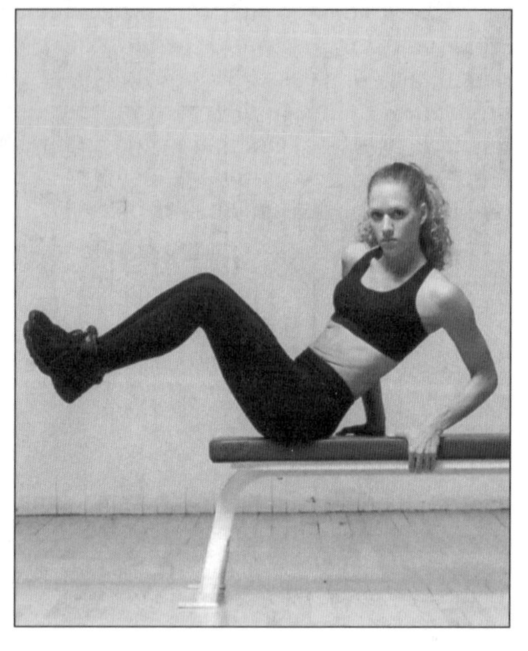

PREPARATION

- Sit on the end of a flat bench.
- Flex hips and knees to 90 degrees.
- Lift feet approximately two to six inches off the floor.
- Place the hands approximately one to two feet behind the buttocks and grasp the sides of the bench, keeping elbows flexed.

ACTION

- Twist the legs to the right.
- Simultaneously "crunch" the upper and lower body, directing the right shoulder toward the left knee.
- Return to the starting position.
- Twist the legs to the left.
- Repeat the movement with the left shoulder directed toward the right knee.

Note: Keep a slight "roll" in the spine. This will help to eliminate hyperextension of the low back.

Roman Chair Side Raise

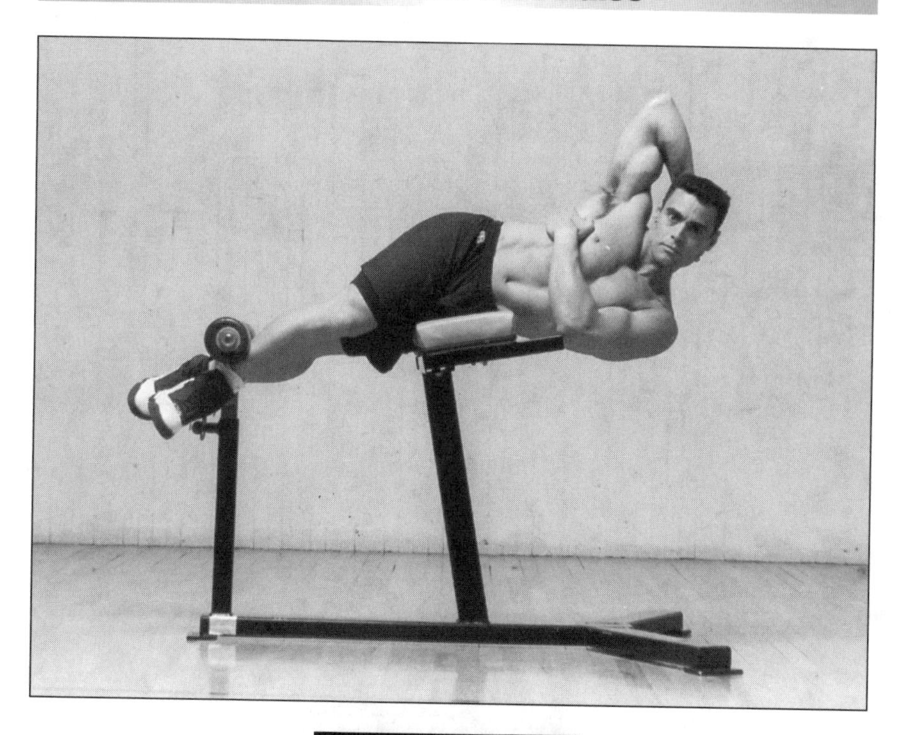

Ab Strength (Obliques)
Slow to Moderate

PREPARATION

- Using a Roman Chair, position the left hip on the front edge of the support pad.
- With the right foot in front of the left, adjust the tibia (lower leg) supports to a comfortable position.
- Place right hand behind the head.
- Place left hand on the working obliques.
- To begin the movement, lean the upper body slightly below horizontal.

ACTION

- Contract the right obliques and raise the upper body to a position slightly above horizontal, avoiding lifting with the legs.
- Direct the right elbow toward the right hip.
- Hold for one count (i.e., "one-thousand-one").
- Slowly return to the starting position.
- Continue on the same side for one set.
- Repeat on the opposite side.

Note: This exercise could possibly cause some discomfort to the low back. We advise caution.

Roman Chair Oblique Twist

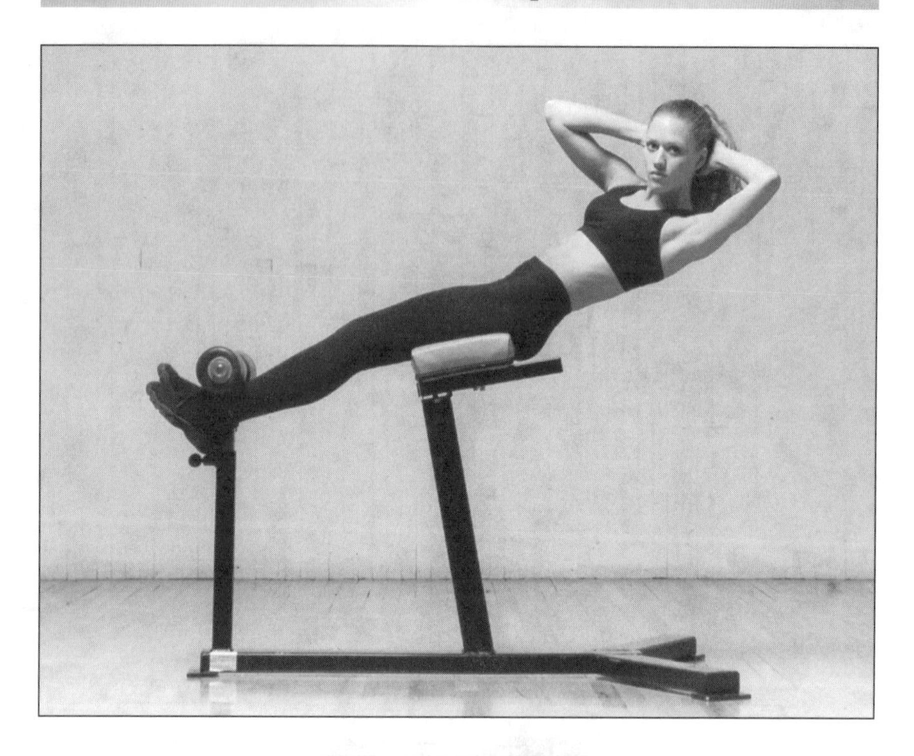

Ab Strength (Obliques)
Moderate

PREPARATION

- Using a Roman Chair, position the ankles under the tibia (lower leg) pads.
- Position hips on the front edge of the torso pad.
- Lean back so the upper body is slightly above horizontal.
- Fold arms across the chest or place hands behind the head.

ACTION

- Isometrically hold the upper body in the extended position.
- Twist to the left.
- The head should "follow" the torso.
- Immediately repeat toward the right.

Note: This exercise could possibly cause some discomfort to the low back. We advise caution. Keep a slight "roll" in the spine. This will help to eliminate hyperextension of the low back.

Roman Chair Oblique Lift and Twist

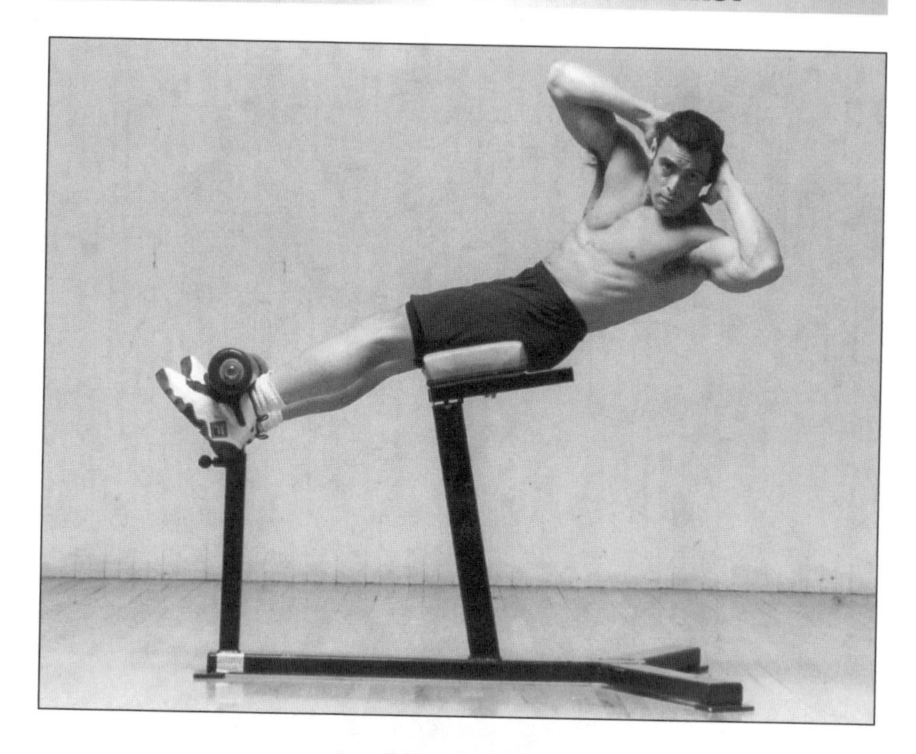

Ab Strength (Obliques)
Moderate

PREPARATION

- Using a Roman Chair, position the ankles under the tibia (lower leg) pads.
- Position hips on the front edge of the torso pad.
- Lean back so the upper body is slightly above horizontal.
- Fold arms across the chest or place hands behind the head.

ACTION

- Isolate the left obliques and upper abs but avoid lifting with the legs.
- Lift and twist the upper body approximately 8 to 12 inches.
- Return to the starting position.
- Either continue to the same side for one set or alternate sides.

Note: This exercise could possibly cause some discomfort to the low back. We advise caution. Keep a slight "roll" in the spine. This will help to eliminate hyper-extension of the low back.

Roman Chair Russian Twist

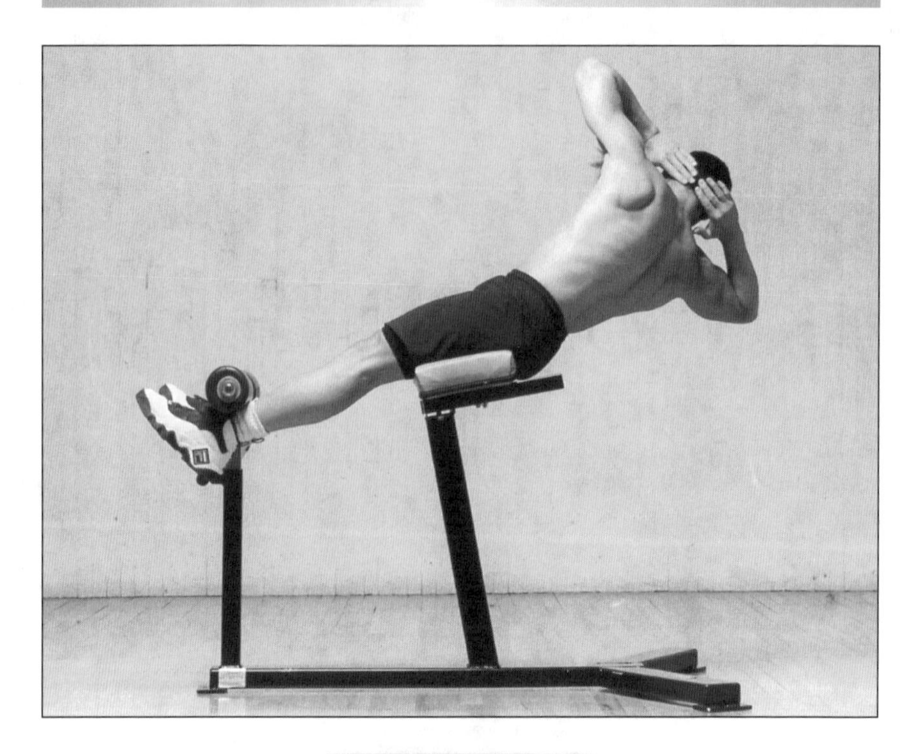

Ab Strength (Obliques)
Slow

PREPARATION

- Using a Roman Chair, position the ankles under the tibia (lower leg) pads.
- Position hips on the front edge of the torso pad.
- Lean back to an angle approximately 45 degrees from the floor.
- Fold arms across the chest or place hands behind the head.

ACTION

- Twist left.
- Drop the upper body six to eight inches.
- Twist right.
- Lift the upper body six to eight inches, avoiding lifting with the legs.
- Continue the same direction for one set.
- Repeat toward the opposite direction.

Note: This exercise could possibly cause some discomfort to the low back. We advise caution. Keep a slight "roll" in the spine. This will help to eliminate hyperextension of the low back.

Freestanding Leg Raise With Oblique Crunch

Ab Strength (Obliques)
Moderate

PREPARATION

- Position the lumbar support pad in the small of the back.
- Rest elbows on the elbow support pads, slightly in front of the upper body.
- Lightly grasp the handles.
- Flex hips and knees to 90 degrees.
- Do not hyperextend the low back.
- With the shoulders square to the apparatus, twist the lower body to the left.

ACTION

- Contract the right obliques and lower abs and lift the legs 8 to 10 inches.
- Avoid "throwing" or using momentum to lift the legs.
- Hold for one count.
- Return to the starting position.
- Continue toward the same side for one set.
- Repeat toward the opposite side.

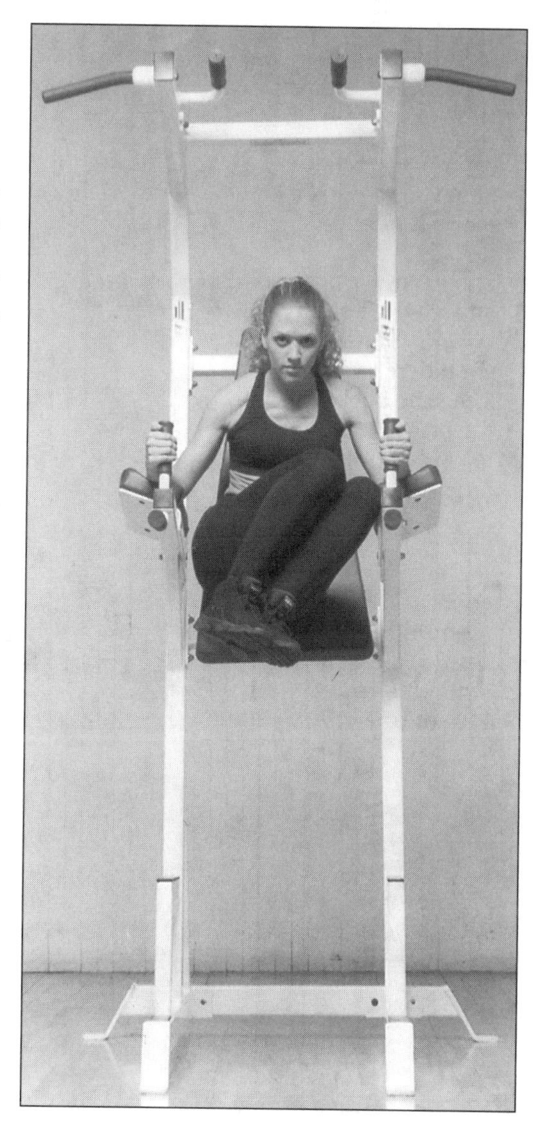

Seated Barbell Twist

Ab Strength (Obliques)
Slow

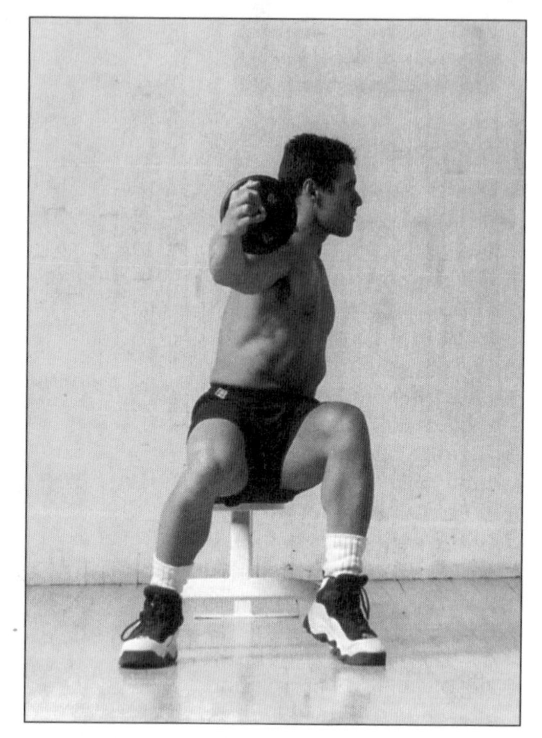

PREPARATION

- Sit on a flat bench.
- Place the feet flat on the floor.
- Start with a broomstick and work up to a light barbell positioned across the shoulders.
- Keep the back straight.
- Keep the head up, focusing eyes straight ahead.

ACTION

- Slowly twist the torso to the left and hold for one count.
- Remember to keep the head up, focusing eyes straight ahead.
- Repeat toward the right.

Barbell Side Bend

Ab Strength (Obliques)
Slow

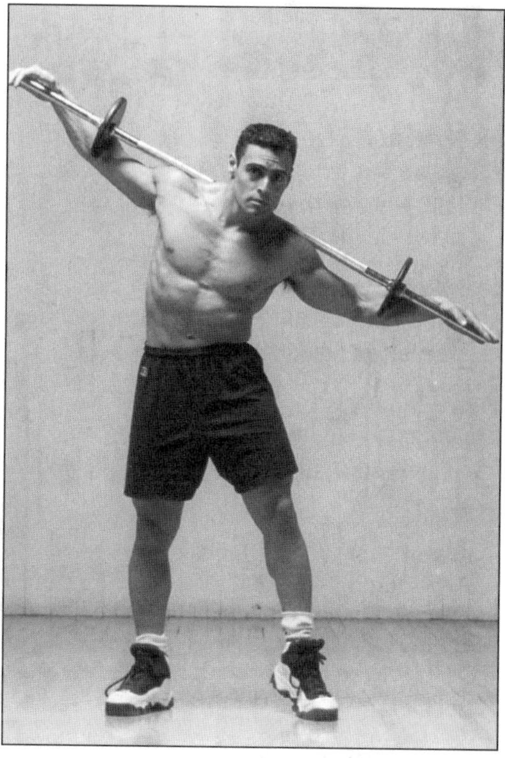

PREPARATION

- Stand erect with feet shoulder-width apart.
- Flex knees slightly.
- Start with a broomstick and work up to a light barbell positioned across the shoulders.
- Keep the back straight.
- Keep the head up, focusing eyes straight ahead.

ACTION

- Contract the left obliques and bend sideways at the waist.
- Isolate the movement at the waist, not at the knees.
- Range of motion is limited, therefore, do not lean too far to the left.
- To ensure a complete "crunch" of the left obliques, simultaneously raise the left heel off the floor.
- Hold for one count.
- Either continue toward the same side for one set or alternate sides.

Note: You can also do this drill while sitting on a flat bench.

Single-Arm Dumbbell Side Bend

Ab Strength (Obliques)
Slow

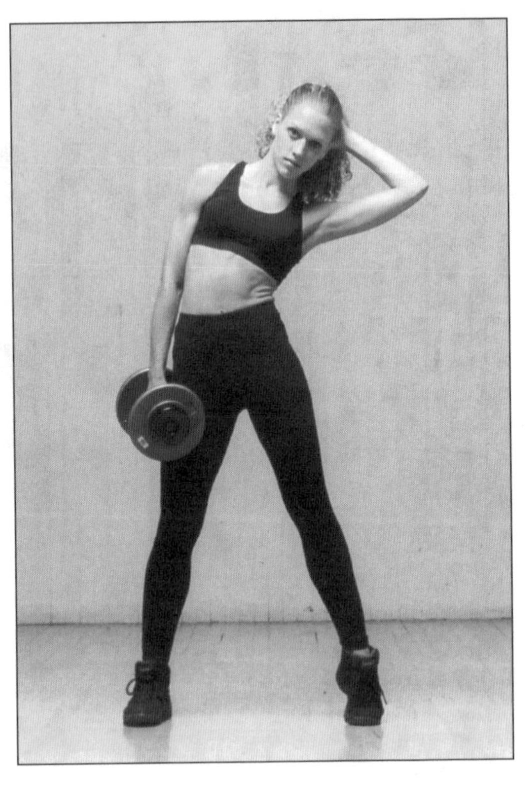

PREPARATION

- Stand erect with feet slightly wider than shoulder-width apart.
- Flex knees slightly.
- Hold a dumbbell in the right hand.
- Place left hand behind the head.
- Keep the back straight.
- Keep the head up, focusing eyes straight ahead.

ACTION

- To start, allow the weight of the dumbbell to pull the upper body slowly to the right.
- Contract the left obliques and pull the weight back to the left.
- Isolate the movement at the waist, not at the knees.
- Range of motion is limited, therefore, do not lean too far to the left.
- To ensure a complete "crunch" of the left obliques, simultaneously raise the left heel off the floor.
- Hold for one count.
- Return to the starting position.
- Continue toward the same side for one set.
- Repeat toward the opposite side.

Note: If you are a beginner, start with no weight at all; you should not use dumbbells until you have mastered the technique of this drill. As you grow stronger, practice with water jugs, phone books, or very light dumbbells before using heavier resistance.

Kneeling Pull-Down Twist

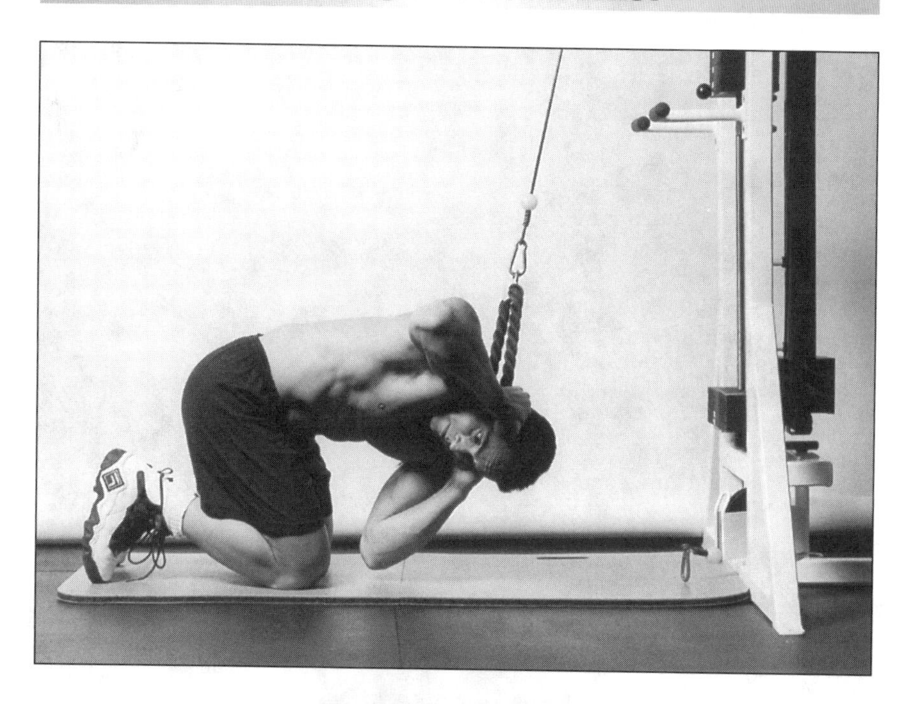

Ab Strength (Obliques)
Slow

PREPARATION

- To begin, select a light weight and only increase the resistance as strength levels and mastery of technique dictate.
- Kneel on the floor in front of a Cable Cross machine (can also be done using some Lat Pull machines).
- Flex knees to 90 degrees, keeping them 8 to 12 inches apart.
- Keep upper body parallel to the floor and back straight. (*Note:* An extension cable supplied by the manufacturer may be necessary for some machinery.)
- Grasp the rope (or bar, or a towel doubled over a bar, or the like) and hold firmly behind the head.

ACTION

- Contract the obliques and pull the left elbow toward the right knee.
- Hold for one count.
- Slowly return to the starting position.
- Either continue toward the same side for one set or alternate sides.

Note: Avoid excessive movement at the hip and hyperextension of the low back. The only movement should be the limited range of motion made by contracting the obliques.

Standing Pull-Down Twist

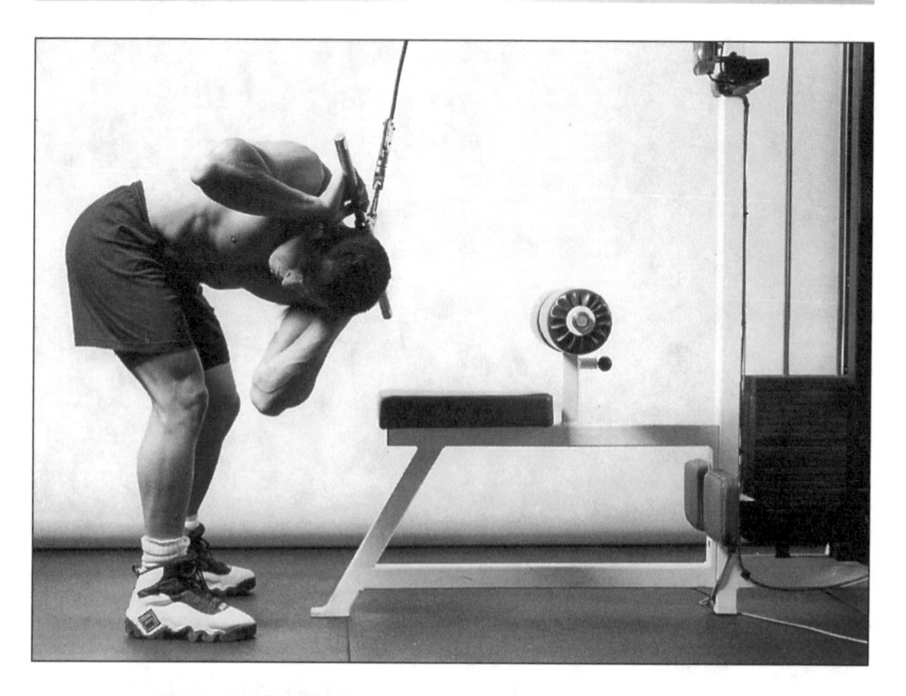

Ab Strength (Obliques)
Slow

PREPARATION

- To begin, select a light weight, only increasing the resistance as strength level and mastery of technique dictate.
- Stand on the floor in front of a Lat Pull machine (can also be done using some Cable Cross machines).
- Slightly flex knees with feet shoulder-width apart.
- Position so that when you bend 90 degrees at the hips, that is, when upper body is parallel to the floor, the bar will be directly above your neck.
- Once the feet are comfortably positioned, reach up and grasp the bar with an overhand grip.
- Lower the upper body to a horizontal position.
- Place the bar behind the head with hands next to the ears.

ACTION

- Contract the obliques and pull the left elbow toward the right knee.
- Hold for one count.
- Slowly return to the starting position.
- Either continue toward the same side for one set or alternate sides.
- Avoid using the muscles of the legs; instead, concentrate on the muscles you're training.

Note: Avoid excessive movement at the hip and hyperextension of the low back. The only movement should be the limited range of motion made by contracting the obliques. You may want to avoid this drill altogether if you are prone to low back injury.

Seated Pull-Down Twist

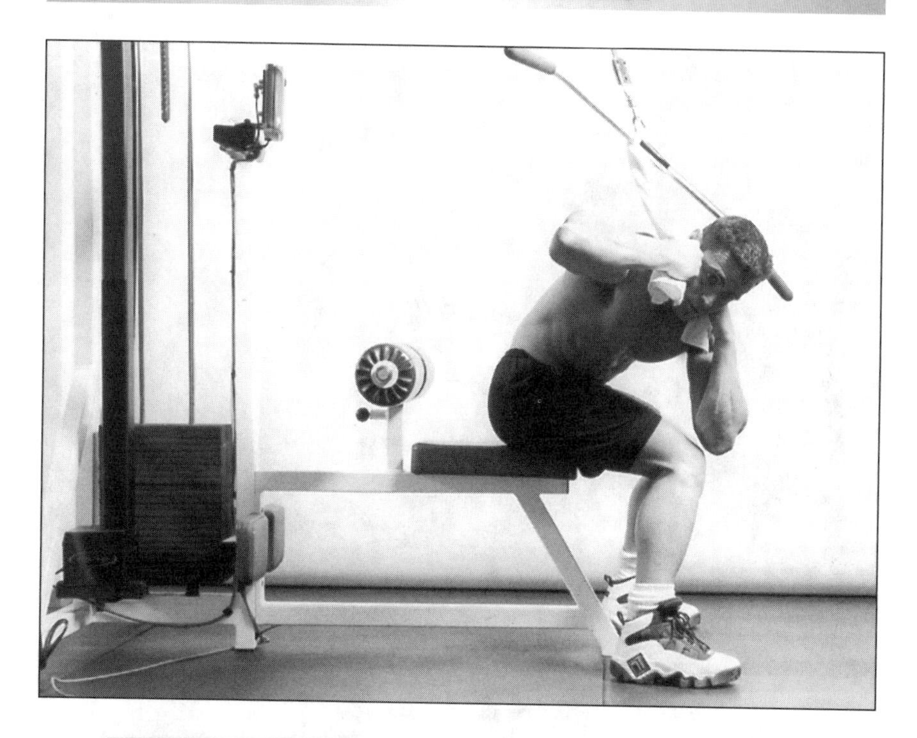

Ab Strength (Obliques)
Slow

PREPARATION

- To begin, select a light weight, only increasing the resistance as strength level and mastery of technique dictate.
- Sit on a Lat Pull machine, keeping back toward the machine.
- Place feet flat on the floor, 12 to 18 inches apart.
- Grasp the rope (or towel) and hold tightly next to the head.
- With the thighs parallel to the floor, lower the upper body to a 45-degree angle.

ACTION

- Contract the obliques and pull the left elbow toward the right knee.
- Hold for one count.
- Slowly return to the starting position.
- Either continue toward the same side for one set or alternate sides.

Note: Avoid excessive movement at the hip and hyperextension of the low back. The only movement should be the limited range of motion made by contracting the obliques.

Vertical Row With Single-Arm Twist

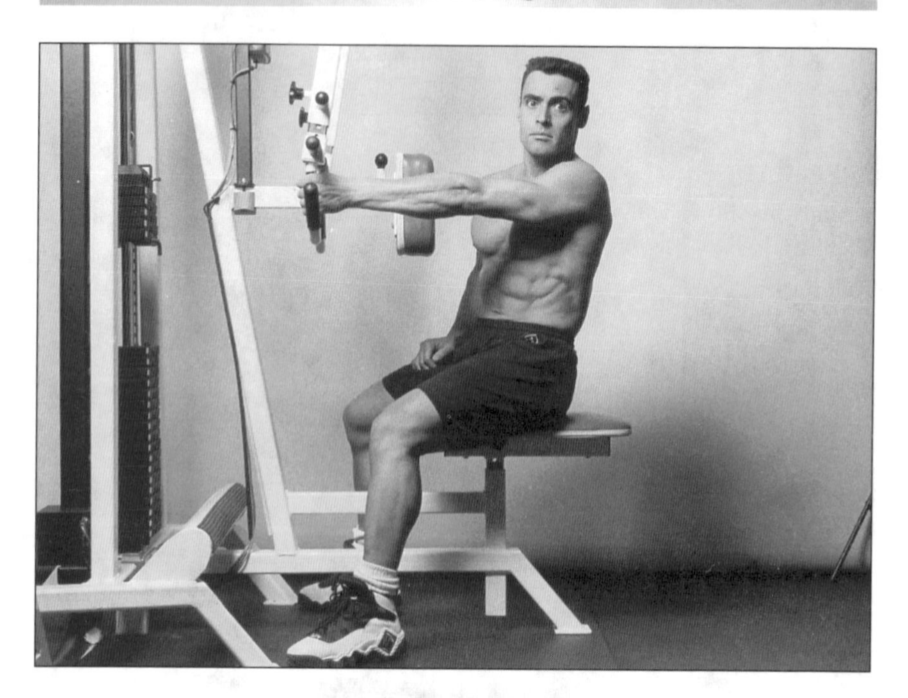

Ab Strength (Obliques)
Slow to Moderate

PREPARATION

- To begin, select a light weight, only increasing the resistance as strength level and mastery of technique dictate.
- Sit at either a Vertical Row or a Low Pulley machine.
- Stabilize the lower body by having a wide base of support with the feet.
- Keep the back straight.
- Grasp the handle with the left hand.
- Keep left arm straight.

ACTION

- Rotate the upper body counterclockwise, pulling the left arm back as far as comfortably possible, while maintaining the correct posture described above.
- Pull with the obliques, not the arms.
- Hold for one count.
- Slowly return to the starting position (do not drop the weight stack).
- Continue toward the same side for one set.
- Repeat toward the opposite side.

Rotary Torso

Ab Strength (Obliques)
Slow

PREPARATION

- Many machines will vary as to the mechanical design.
- Follow the guidelines suggested by the manufacturer.

ACTION

- Follow the manufacturer's directions for the exercise.

Flat Bench Knee-Ups

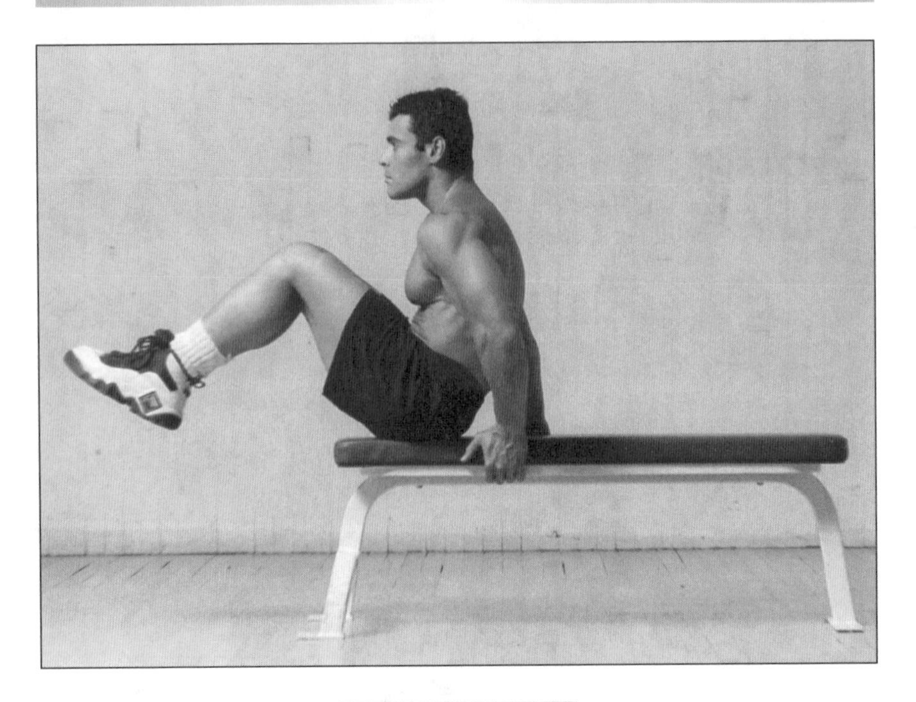

Ab Strength (Lower)
Moderate

PREPARATION

- Sit on the end of a flat bench.
- Keep legs straight with knees slightly flexed.
- Lift feet approximately two to six inches off the floor.
- Place the hands approximately one to two feet behind the buttocks and grasp the sides of the bench, keeping elbows flexed.

ACTION

- Bend the knees and lift toward the upper body, while the upper body simultaneously "crunches" toward the knees.
- Return to the starting position.
- Immediately repeat.

Note: Keep a slight "roll" in the spine. This will help to eliminate hyperextension of the low back.

Flat Bench Straight Leg Lifts

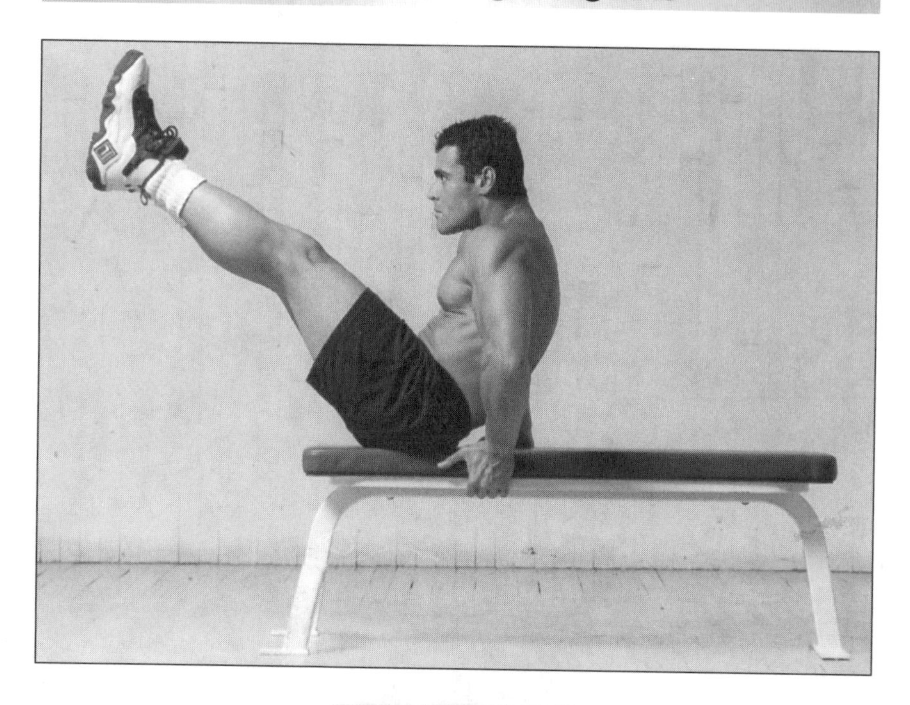

Ab Strength (Lower)
Moderate

PREPARATION

- Sit on the end of a bench.
- Keep legs straight with knees slightly flexed.
- Lift feet approximately two to six inches off the floor.
- Place the hands approximately one to two feet behind the buttocks and grasp the sides of the bench, keeping elbows flexed.

ACTION

- Lift straight legs and upper body simultaneously toward a "pike" position.
- Return to the starting position.
- Immediately repeat.

Note: Keep a slight "roll" in the spine. This will help to eliminate hyperextension of the low back.

Slant Board Knee-Ups

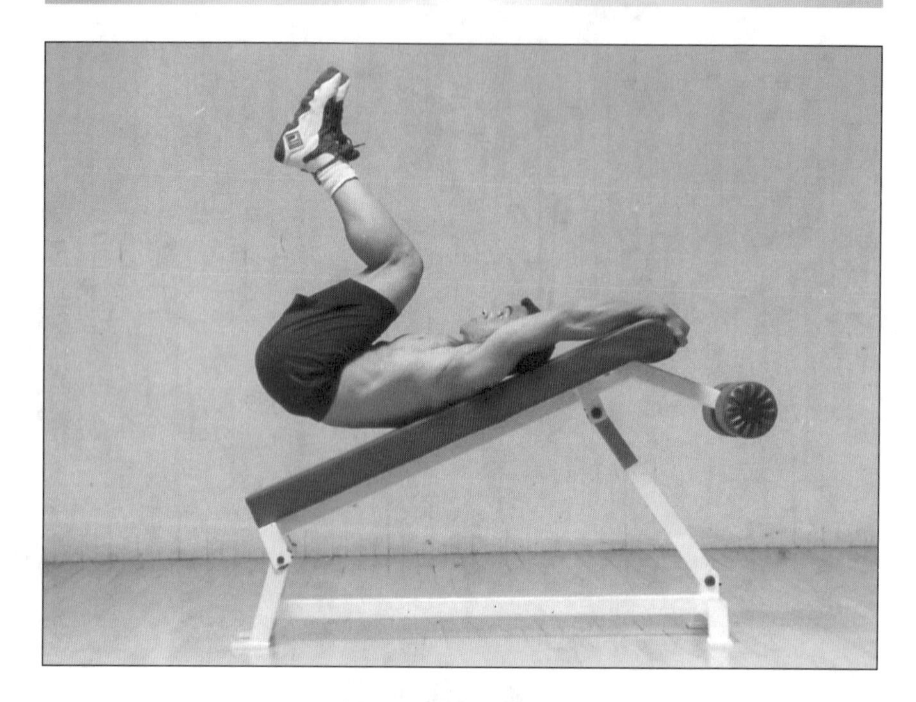

Ab Strength (Lower)
Slow

PREPARATION

- Adjust the sit-up board to a challenging angle within a range of 15 degrees for beginners to 30 degrees for advanced exercisers.
- Lie on the bench, head toward the top, feet at the bottom.
- Tuck chin to the chest.
- Keep arms straight and extended overhead.
- Grasp the top of the bench (or the support bars, handles, or the like).
- Bend the knees fully.
- Flex the hips so that the upper thighs are resting on the stomach.

ACTION

- Keep the upper spine in contact with the board during the entire set.
- Contract the lower abs to lift the hips six to eight inches *up* and *back*. Isolate the lower abs; do not use momentum from throwing the legs.
- Touch the knees to the armpits.
- Slowly roll back to the starting position.
- Immediately repeat.

Note: Do not pull with the arms. Keep them relatively straight throughout the exercise.

Slant Board Leg Thrust

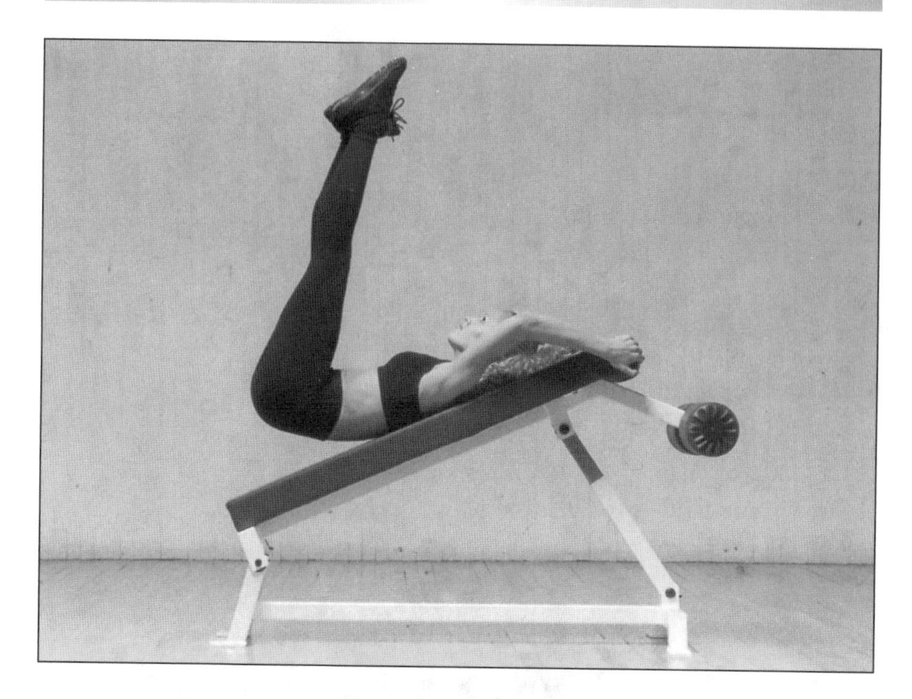

Ab Strength (Lower)
Moderate

PREPARATION

- Adjust the sit-up board to a challenging angle within a range of 15 degrees for beginners to 30 degrees for advanced exercisers.
- Lie on the bench, head toward the top, feet at the bottom.
- Keep the head back, chin should not touch the chest.
- Keep arms straight and extended overhead.
- Grasp the top of the bench (or the support bar, handles, or the like).
- Lift the hips and point the toes to the ceiling.
- Keep legs straight and perpendicular to the ceiling throughout the exercise.

ACTION

- Thrust the legs straight up toward the ceiling, not back over the face.
- Slowly return to the starting position.
- Immediately repeat.

Note: Do not pull with the arms. Keep them relatively straight throughout the exercise.

Freestanding Leg Raise—Bent-Knee

Ab Strength (Lower)
Moderate

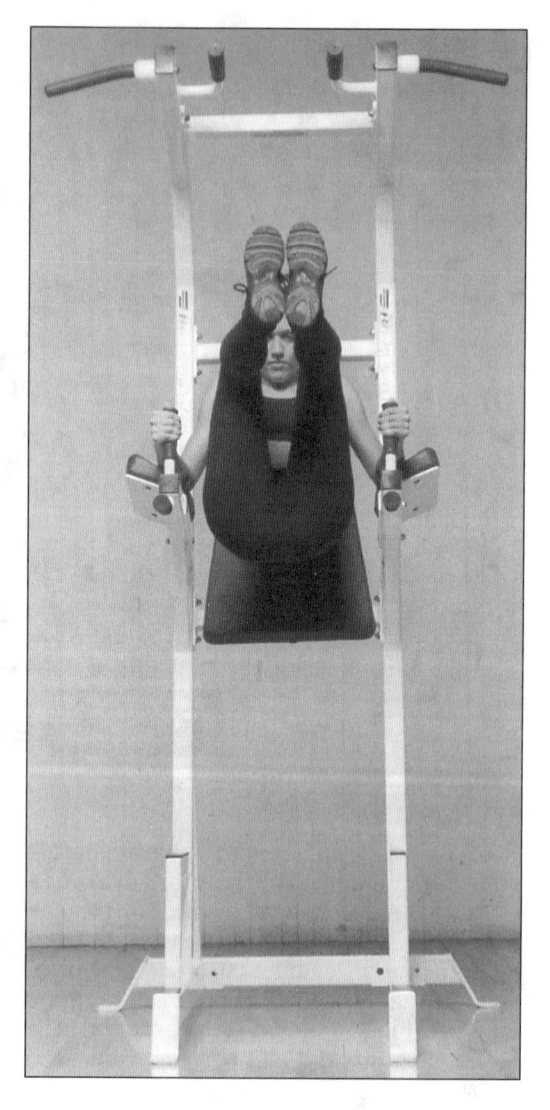

PREPARATION

- Position the lumbar support in the small of the back.
- Keep the head forward, focusing eyes straight ahead.
- Rest elbows on the elbow support pads, slightly in front of the upper body.
- Lightly grasp the handles.
- Flex hips and knees to 90 degrees.
- Do not hyperextend the low back.

ACTION

- Isolate the lower abs and lift (roll back) the knees toward the chest. Hips should lift off the lumbar support pad.
- Slowly lower the legs to the starting position.
- Do not drop the legs below the starting position.
- Immediately repeat.

Note: Range of motion should be limited. Do not throw the legs to generate momentum.

Freestanding Leg Raise—Alternating Straight Leg

Ab Strength (Lower)
Moderate

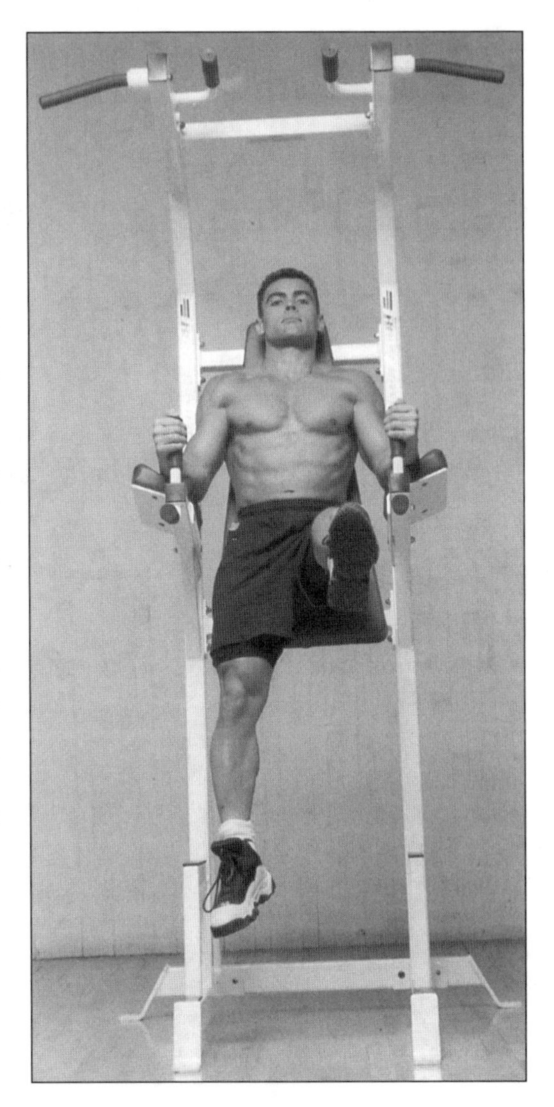

PREPARATION

- Position the lumbar support in the small of the back.
- Keep the head forward, focusing eyes straight ahead.
- Rest elbows on the elbow support pads, slightly in front of the upper body.
- Lightly grasp the handles.
- Extend both legs toward the floor.
- Do not hyperextend the low back.

ACTION

- Lift the left leg to horizontal (right leg remains down).
- Return to the starting position.
- Repeat with the opposite leg.

Freestanding Leg Raise—Straight Leg

Ab Strength (Lower)
Moderate

PREPARATION

- Position the lumbar support in the small of the back.
- Keep the head forward, focusing eyes straight ahead.
- Rest elbows on the elbow support pads, slightly in front of the upper body.
- Lightly grasp the handles.
- Extend both legs toward the floor.
- Do not hyperextend the low back.

ACTION

- In a controlled manner, lift both legs to horizontal (90-degree angle at the hip).
- Slowly return to the starting position.
- Immediately repeat.

Note: As strength levels improve, try lifting the legs to a position above horizontal (as pictured here).

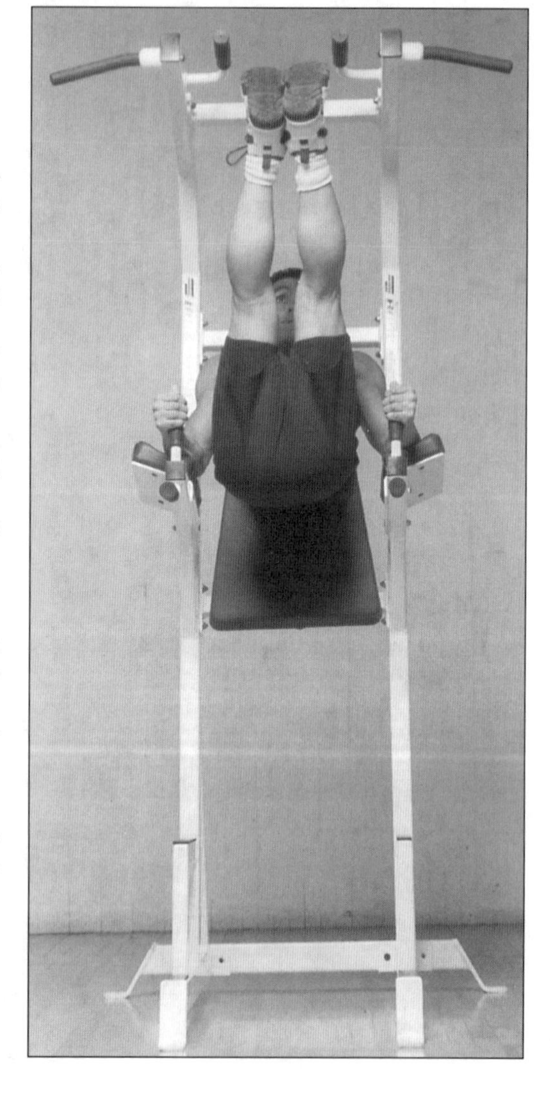

Hanging Curl

Ab Strength (Lower)
Moderate

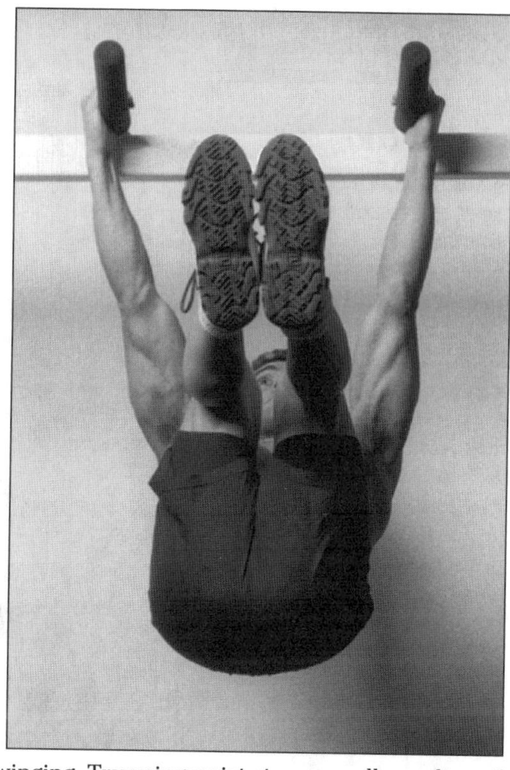

PREPARATION

- Grasp a chin-up bar slightly wider than shoulder-width apart.
- Flex hips and knees to 90 degrees.

ACTION

- Isolating the lower abs, curl the knees back toward the armpits, avoiding pulling up with the arms.
- Slowly return to the starting position, avoiding swinging.
- Do not allow the legs to drop below the starting position.
- Immediately repeat.

Note: This exercise works best if a partner stands behind and helps keep the exerciser from swinging. Try using wrist straps or elbow slings if shoulder and arm strength are inadequate to maintain correct technique.

Hanging Pike

Ab Strength (Lower)
Moderate

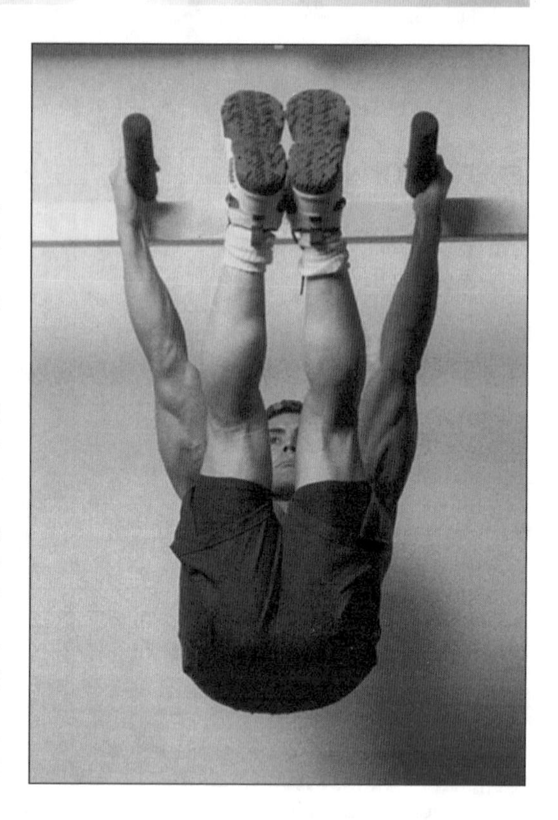

PREPARATION

- Grasp a chin-up bar slightly wider than shoulder-width apart.
- Hang legs straight with knees slightly flexed.

ACTION

- Isolate the lower abs and lift both legs simultaneously.
- Tap the feet to the bar.
- Do not hyperextend the low back or use a preparatory swing to gain assistance from momentum.
- Maintain a "hunch" or "curve" in the back during the lift.
- Slowly return to the starting position, avoiding swinging.
- Immediately repeat.

Note: This drill requires considerable abdominal strength and coordination. This exercise works best if a partner stands behind and helps keep the exerciser from swinging. Try using wrist straps or elbow slings if shoulder and arm strength are inadequate to maintain correct technique.

Kneeling Pull-Down Crunch

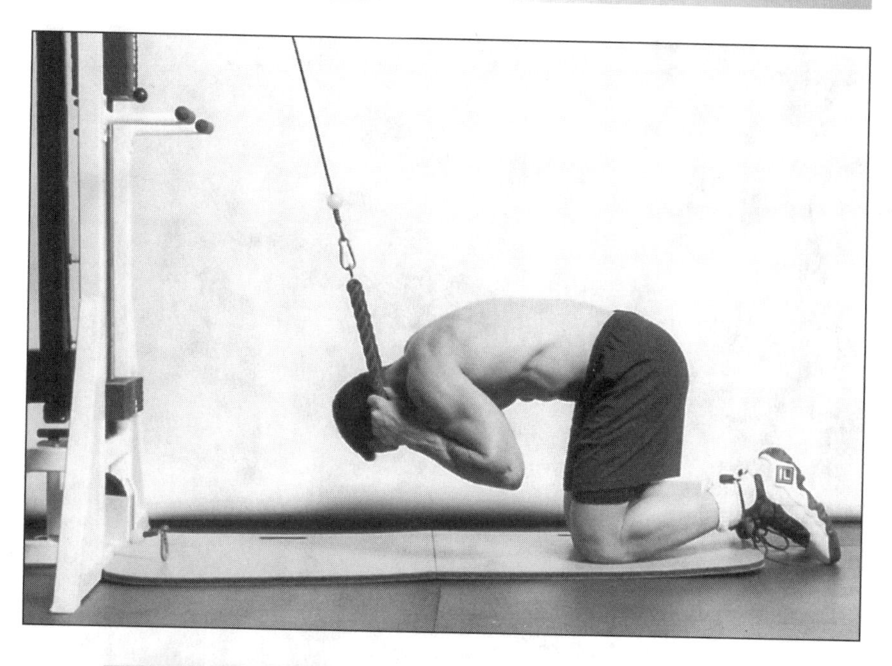

Ab Strength (Upper)
Slow

PREPARATION

- To begin, select a light weight, only increasing the resistance as strength level and mastery of technique dictate.
- Kneel on the floor in front of a Cable Cross machine (can also be done using some Lat Pull machines).
- Flex knees to 90 degrees, holding them 8 to 12 inches apart.
- Keep upper body parallel to the floor and the back straight. (*Note*: An extension cable supplied by the manufacturer may be necessary for some machinery.)
- Grasp the rope (or bar, or a towel doubled over a bar, or the like) and hold firmly behind the head.

ACTION

- Contract the upper abs and "curl" the shoulders down toward the floor.
- Move elbows toward the thighs.
- Hold for one count.
- Slowly return to the starting position.
- Immediately repeat.

Note: Avoid excessive movement at the hips and hyperextension of the low back. The only movement should be the limited range of motion made by contracting the upper abs.

Standing Pull-Down Crunch

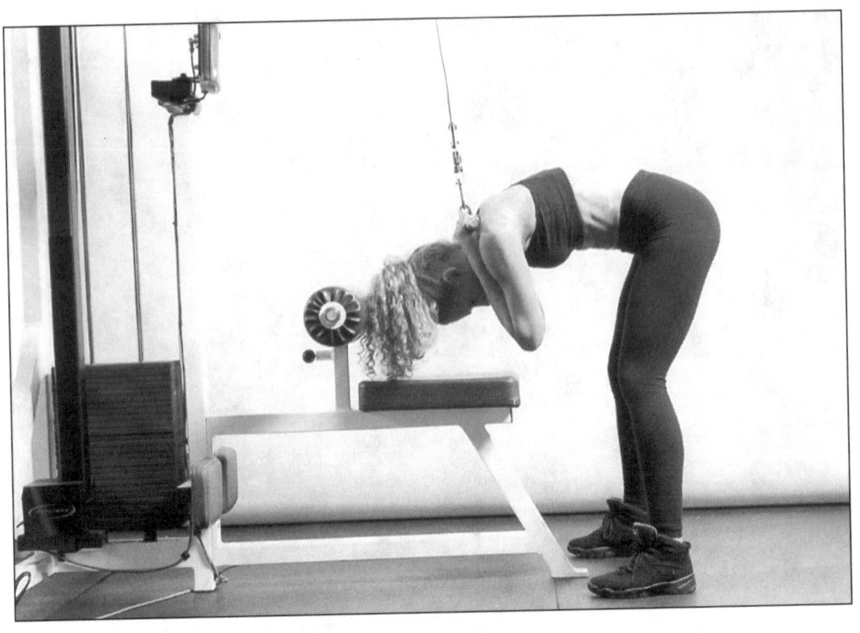

Ab Strength (Upper)
Slow

PREPARATION

- To begin, select a light weight, only increasing the resistance as strength level and mastery of technique dictate.
- Stand on the floor in front of a Lat Pull machine (can also be done using some Cable Cross machines).
- Keep legs straight with feet shoulder-width apart.
- Position so that when you flex 90 degrees at the hips, that is, when upper body is parallel to the floor, the bar will be directly above your neck.
- Once the feet are comfortably positioned, reach up and grasp the bar with an underhand grip.
- Lower the upper body to a horizontal position.
- Place the bar behind the head with hands next to the ears.

ACTION

- Contract the upper abs and curl the shoulders.
- Move elbows toward the thighs.
- Hold for one count.
- Slowly return to the starting position.
- Immediately repeat.

Note: Avoid excessive movement at the hip and hyperextension of the low back. The only movement should be the limited range of motion made by contracting the upper abs. This exercise could possibly cause some discomfort to the low back. We advise caution.

Seated Pull-Down Crunch

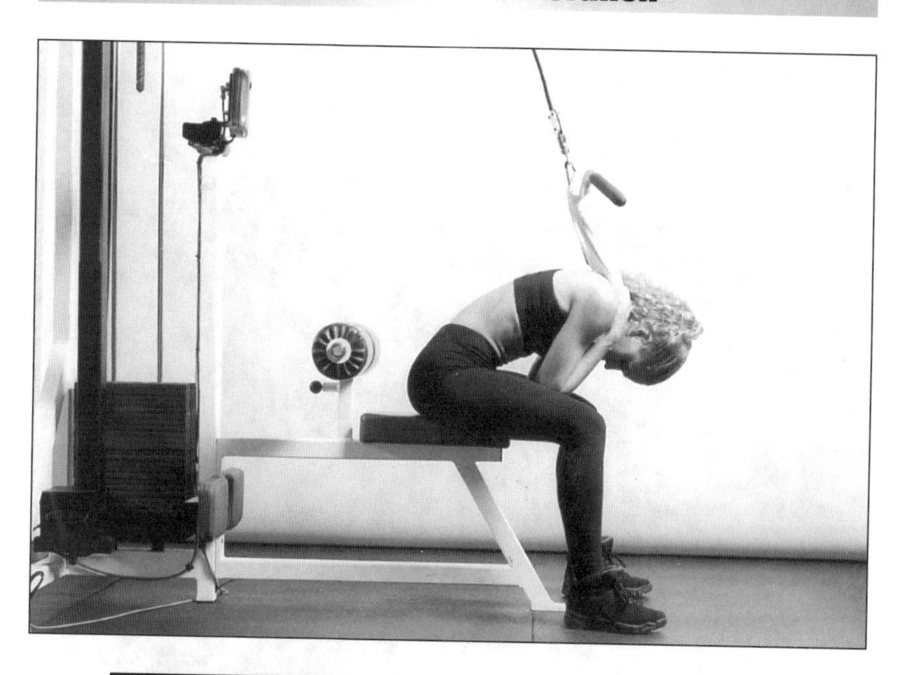

Ab Strength (Upper)
Slow

PREPARATION

- To begin, select a light weight, only increasing the resistance as strength level and mastery of technique dictate.
- Sit on a Lat Pull machine with back toward the machine.
- Place feet flat on the floor, 12 to 18 inches apart.
- Grasp the rope (or bar, or a towel doubled over a bar, or the like) and hold tightly next to the head.
- With the thighs parallel to the floor, lower the upper body to a 45-degree angle.

ACTION

- Contract the upper abs and "curl" the shoulders.
- Move elbows toward the thighs.
- Hold for one count.
- Slowly return to the starting position.
- Immediately repeat.

Note: Avoid excessive movement at the hip and hyperextension of the low back. The only movement should be the limited range of motion made by contracting the upper abs.

Roman Chair Upper Ab Isolate

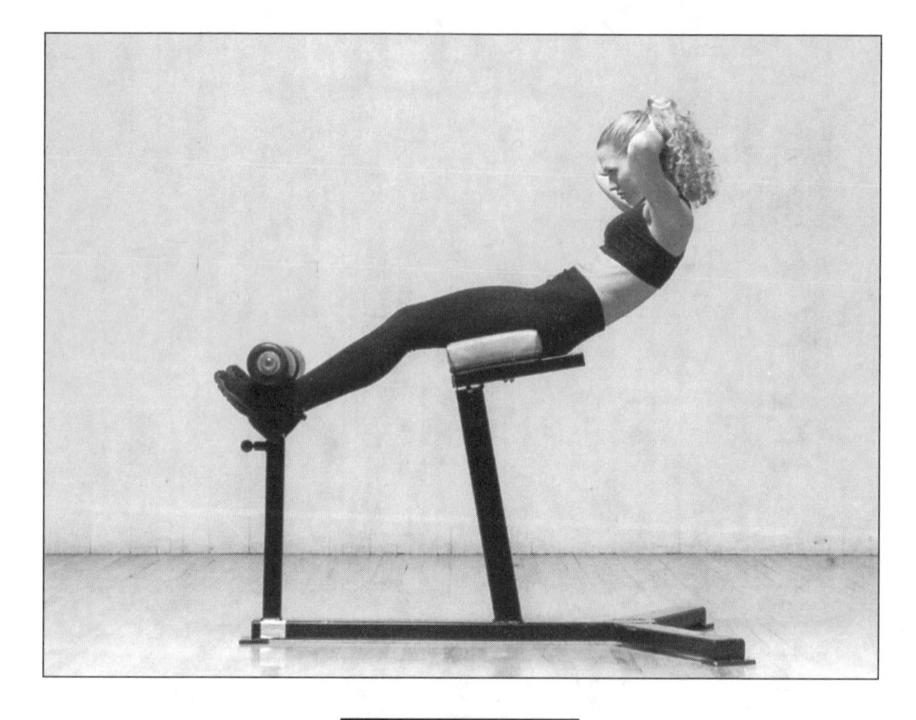

Ab Strength (Upper)
Slow to Moderate

PREPARATION

- Using a Roman Chair, position the ankles under the tibia (lower leg) pads.
- Position hips on the front edge of the torso pad.
- Lean back to where the upper body is slightly above horizontal. Hold this position by isometrically contracting the lower abs and hip flexor muscles.
- Fold arms across the chest or place hands behind the head.

ACTION

- Contract the upper abs and roll the shoulders forward. Do not lift with the muscles of the legs or the lower abdominals.
- Hold for one count.
- Slowly return to the starting position.
- Immediately repeat.

Note: This exercise could possibly cause some discomfort to the low back. We advise caution. Keep a slight "roll" in the spine. This will help to eliminate hyperextension of the low back.

Upper Ab Crunch Machine

Ab Strength (Upper)
Slow to Moderate

PREPARATION

- Machines will vary as to the mechanical design.
- Follow the guidelines suggested by the manufacturer.

ACTION

- Follow the manufacturer's directions for the exercise.

Prone Leg Raise on Table

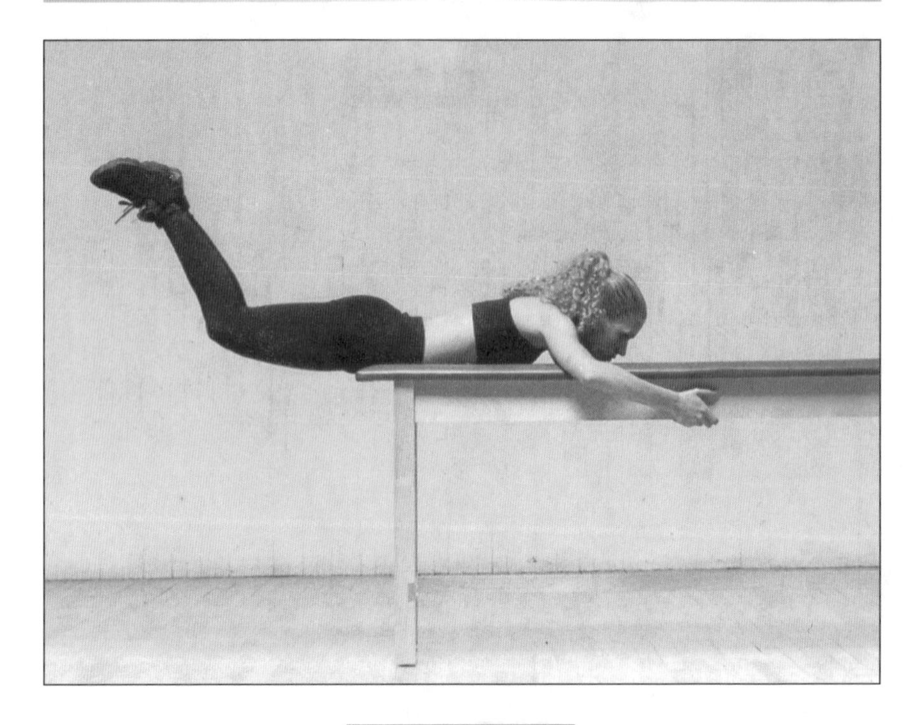

Ab Strength (Back)
Slow

PREPARATION

- Lie on the stomach on a table or flat bench.
- Position the hips on the edge.
- Grasp the sides of the table with the hands.
- Extend legs, knees slightly flexed and flared out, heels touching.

ACTION

- To begin, position legs slightly below parallel to the floor.
- Contract the low back and gluteal muscles.
- Lift the legs to a position above parallel to the floor.
- Hold for several counts.
- Slowly return to the starting position.
- Immediately repeat.

Roman Chair Back Crunch

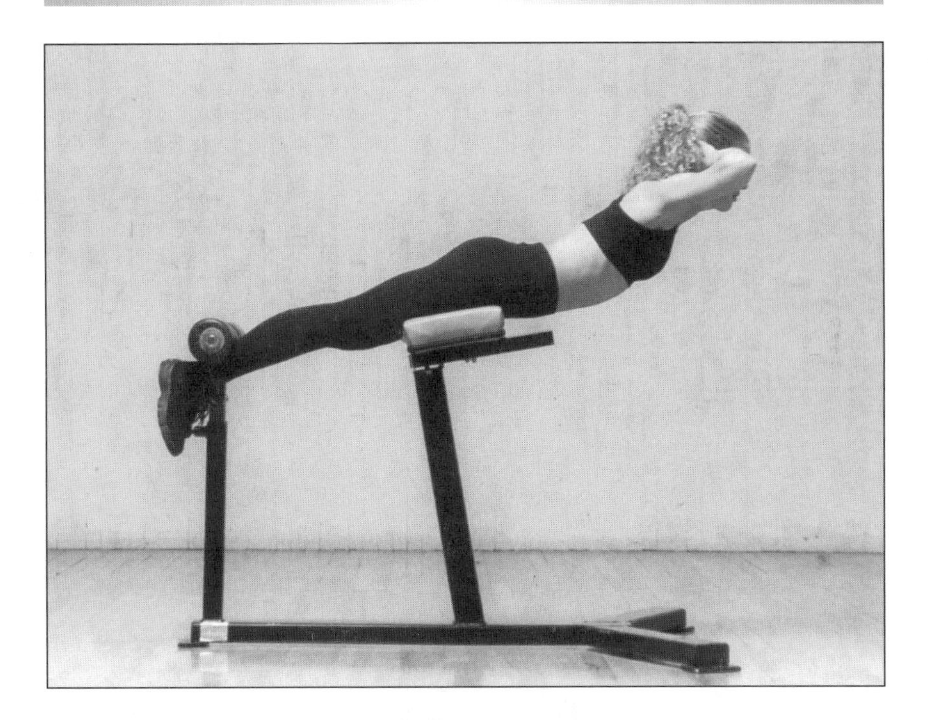

Ab Strength (Back)
Moderate

PREPARATION

- Lying on the stomach, position the body on the Roman Chair with the ankle supports (tibia or lower leg pads) properly adjusted and the hips on the torso pad.
- Bend down at the waist.
- Keep upper body approximately perpendicular to the floor.
- Fold arms across the chest or place hands behind the head.

ACTION

- Contract the low back and gluteal muscles to raise the torso to a position slightly higher than parallel to the floor.
- Hold for one count.
- Slowly return to the starting position.
- Pause for one count (do not bounce at the bottom to gain momentum).
- Immediately repeat.

Note: Inhale while rising, exhale when lowering.

Back Crunch Twist on Roman Chair

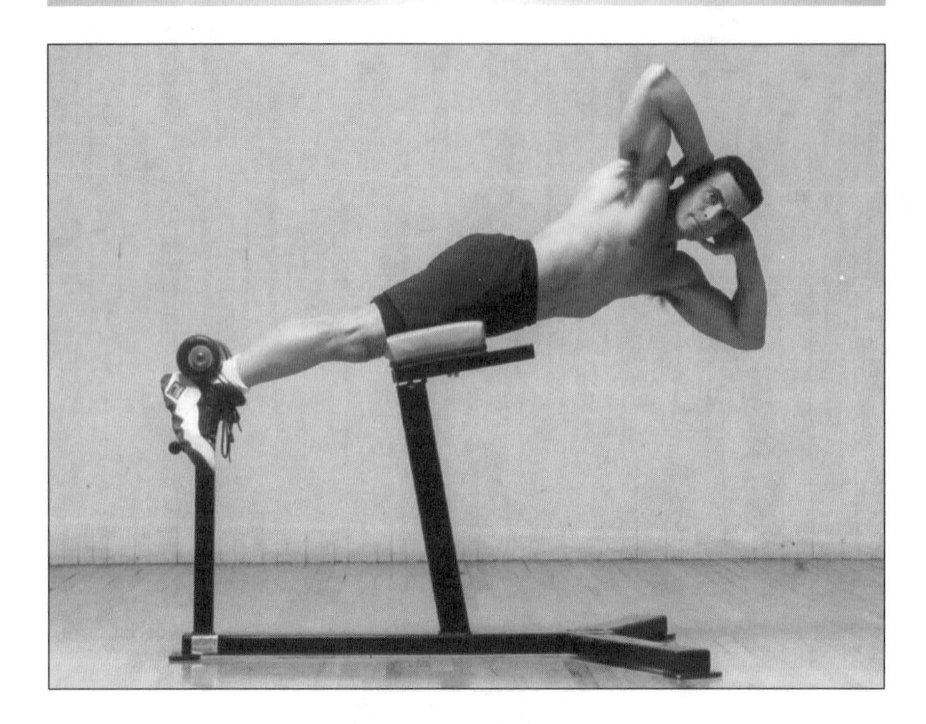

Ab Strength (Back)
Moderate

PREPARATION

- Lying on the stomach, position the body on the Roman Chair with the ankle supports (tibia or lower leg pads) properly adjusted and the hips on the torso pad.
- Bend down at the waist.
- Keep upper body approximately perpendicular to the floor.
- Fold arms across the chest or place hands behind the head.

ACTION

- Contract the low back and gluteal muscles to raise the torso.
- Twist to the left as the torso is rising.
- Stop when the upper torso reaches a position slightly higher than parallel to the floor.
- Hold for one count.
- Slowly return to the starting position.
- Hold for one count (do not bounce at the bottom to gain momentum).
- Repeat toward the right side.

Note: Inhale while rising, exhale when lowering.

Seated Low Pull

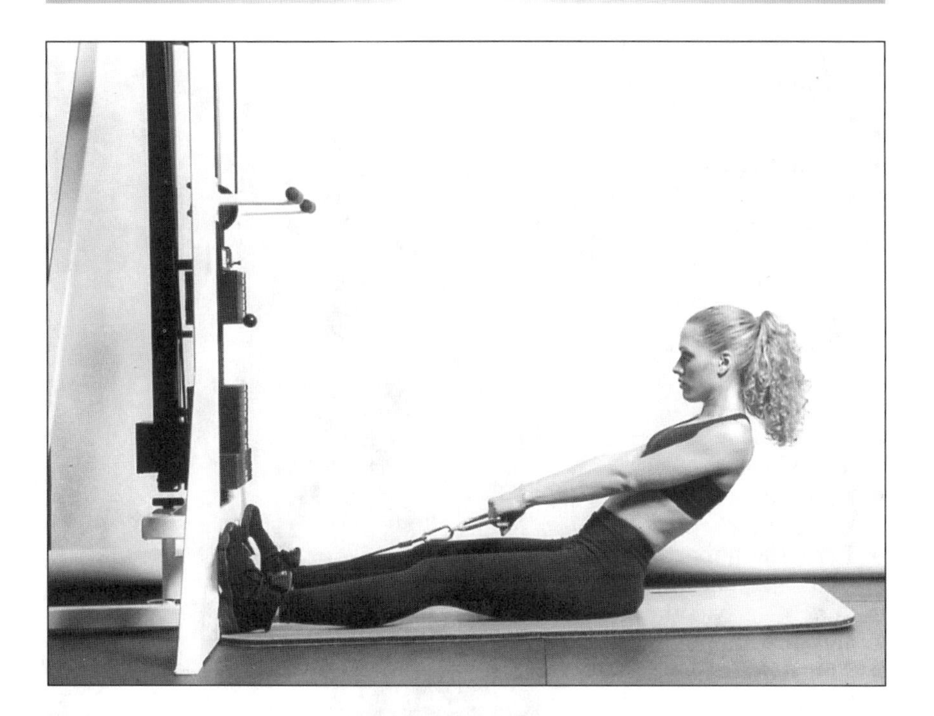

Ab Strength (Back)
Moderate

PREPARATION

- To begin, select a light weight, only increasing the resistance as strength level and mastery of technique dictate.
- Sit on the Low Pulley machine seat (or floor) and place the feet on a support.
- With knees flexed, reach forward and grasp the handles.
- Keep arms straight throughout the exercise.

ACTION

- In a smooth motion, contract the low back muscles and lean back (do not pull with the arms).
- Stop when the upper body is angled approximately 45 degrees to the floor.
- Slowly return to the starting position.
- Immediately repeat.

Midpulley Lumber Rotation

Ab Strength (Back)
Moderate

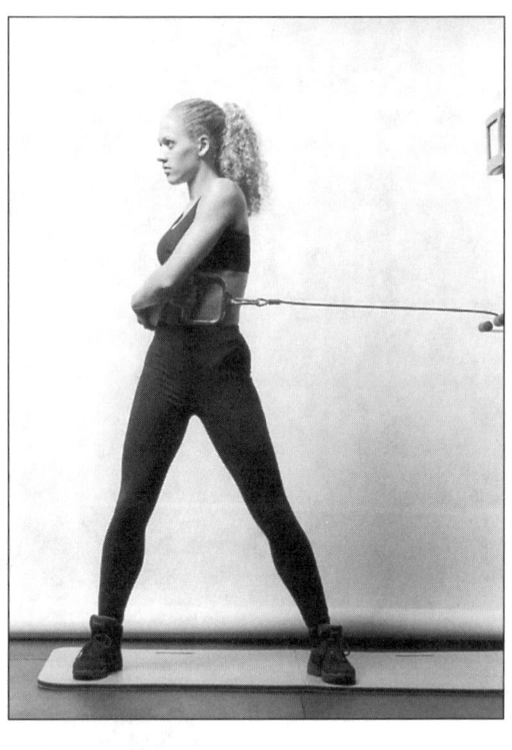

PREPARATION

- To begin, select a light weight, only increasing the resistance as strength level and mastery of technique dictate.
- Stand with your feet shoulder-width apart and perpendicular to the pulley bar, left shoulder closest to the machine.
- Keep the back straight, knees slightly flexed.
- Twist the upper body toward the pulley machine.
- Reach across the body and grip the handle with your right hand.
- Keep your right elbow bent at approximately 90 degrees
- Hold on to your right elbow with your left hand.

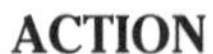

ACTION

- Rotate the trunk and torso to the right.
- Hold for one count.
- Slowly return to the starting position.
- Continue to the same side for one set.
- Repeat toward the opposite side.

Note: While the obliques contribute, the primary muscle involvement will be from the low back.

Low Pulley Diagonal Rotation

Ab Strength (Back)
Moderate

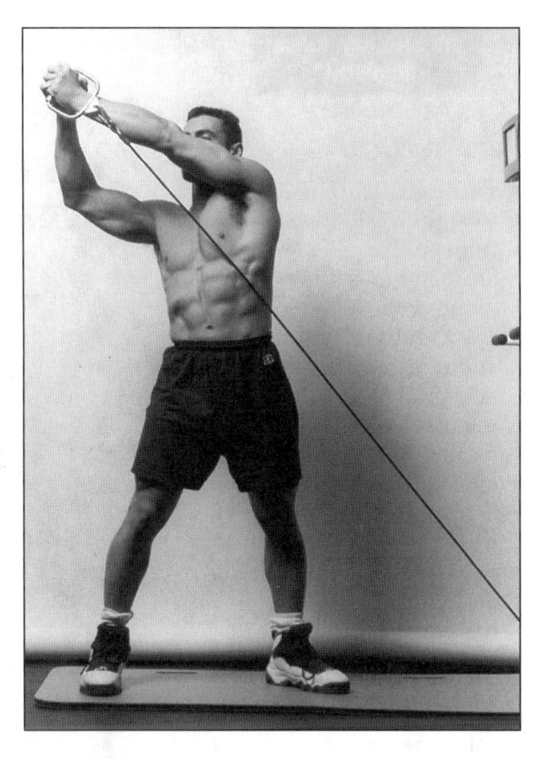

PREPARATION

- To begin, select a light weight, only increasing the resistance as strength level and mastery of technique dictate.
- Stand with your feet shoulder-width apart and perpendicular to the pulley cable, left shoulder closest to the machine.
- Flex knees slightly.
- Twist the upper body toward the pulley machine.
- Reach down with both hands and grasp the low pulley handle.

ACTION

- In one smooth movement, rotate the torso, straighten the back, and pull diagonally across the body (the cable should cross close to the chest).
- Reach as high as comfortably possible.
- Slowly return to the starting position.
- Continue toward the same side for one set.
- Repeat toward the opposite side.

Note: We advise caution for individuals with a history of low back pain or prior injury.

High Pulley Diagonal Rotation

Ab Strength (Back)
Moderate

PREPARATION

- To begin, select a light weight, only increasing the resistance as strength level and mastery of technique dictate.
- Stand tall with your feet shoulder-width apart and perpendicular to the pulley cable, left shoulder closest to the machine.
- Flex knees slightly.
- Twist the upper body toward the pulley machine.
- Reach up with both hands and grasp the high pulley handle.

ACTION

- In one smooth movement, rotate the torso and pull diagonally down across the body (the cable should cross close to the chest and left shoulder).
- Slowly return to the starting position.
- Continue toward the same side for one set.
- Repeat toward the opposite side.

Note: We advise caution for individuals with a history of low back pain or prior injury.

Low Pulley Hip Extension

Ab Strength (Back)
Moderate to Fast

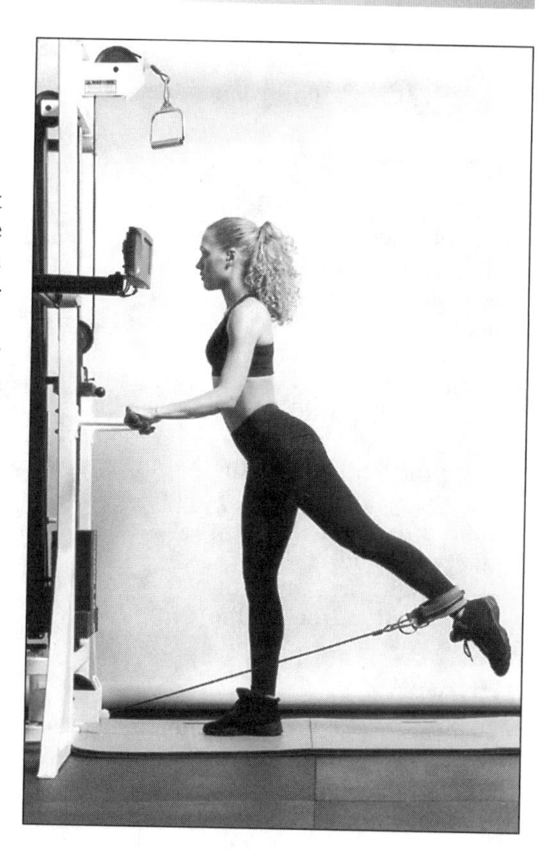

PREPARATION

- To begin, select a light weight, only increasing the resistance as strength level and mastery of technique dictate.
- Stand facing the Low Pulley machine.
- Position the ankle strap on the left ankle.
- Place the hands on the handles or the machine frame away from all moving parts.
- Keep body alignment straight.

ACTION

- Keeping the left leg straight, fully extend the hip backward.
- Hold for one count (do not bounce or jerk to gain momentum).
- Stand tall (do not bend at the waist).
- Slowly return to the starting position.
- Continue for one set.
- Repeat on the opposite side.

Dumbbell Cross Bend

Ab Strength (Back)
Slow to Moderate

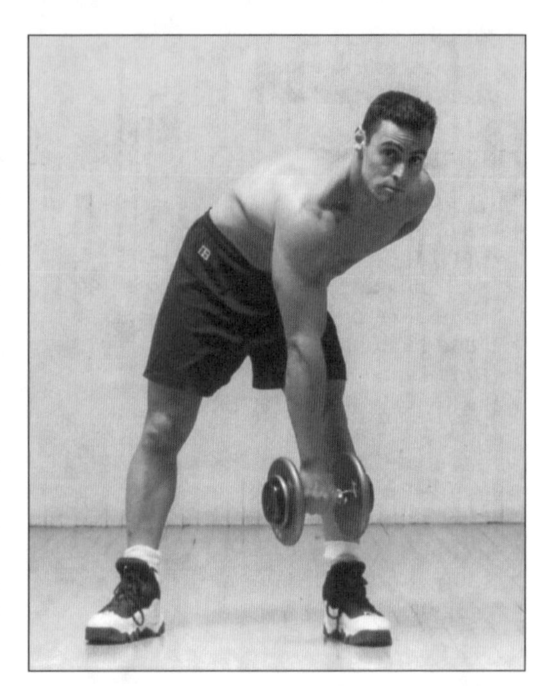

PREPARATION

- To begin, select a light weight, only increasing the resistance as strength level and mastery of technique dictate.
- Stand tall.
- Place feet slightly wider than shoulder-width apart.
- Flex knees slightly.
- Place the left hand on the left hip.
- Hold a light dumbbell in the right hand.
- Keep right arm straight, positioned in front of the body.

ACTION

- Bend and twist so that the dumbbell nearly taps the left thigh. (As strength levels improve, tap the knee, shin, and—ultimately—the foot.)
- Isolating the low back muscles, slowly raise to the starting position.
- Continue toward the same side for one set.
- Repeat toward the opposite side.

Note: We advise caution for individuals with a history of low back pain or prior injury.

Bent-Knee Dead Lift With Barbell

Ab Strength (Back)
Slow

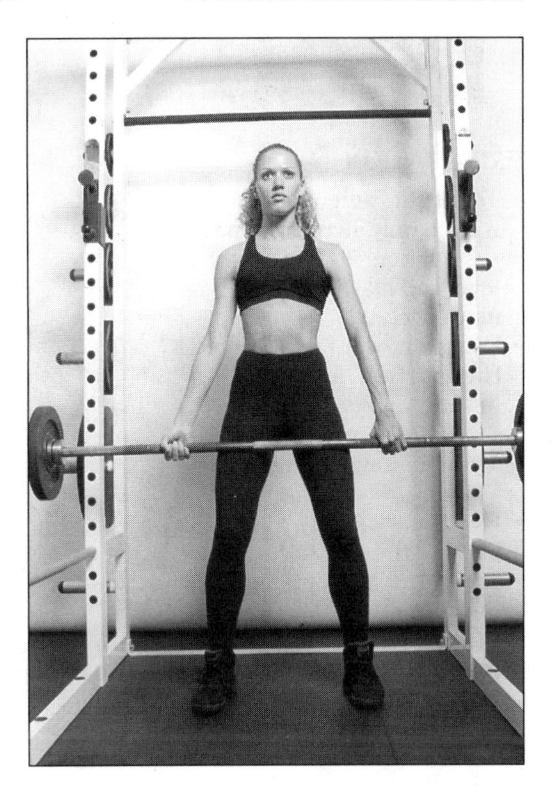

PREPARATION

- To begin, select a light weight, only increasing the resistance as strength level and mastery of technique dictate.
- Using a power rack, place the barbell at slightly lower than knee level.
- Place feet shoulder-width apart.
- Flex knees slightly.
- Bend at the waist.
- Grasp the bar outside of the knees.
- Use an over-under grip (one palm faces forward and the other faces back) to prevent the bar from rolling.
- Keep the back straight.
- Keep the head up.

ACTION

- Start the movement by lifting with the legs.
- Continue the movement by contracting the low back muscles and gluteals, standing erect (do not hyperextend or arch the low back).
- Keep the back straight and the back musculature "tight" throughout the movement.
- Keep legs straight at the top of the movement.
- Keep arms straight and the bar close to the body throughout the lift.
- Slowly return to the starting position by first flexing at the knees, then the hips.
- Immediately repeat (do not bounce or jerk the bar to gain momentum).

Note: We advise caution for individuals with a history of low back pain or injury. Inhale up, exhale down. You can also do this exercise using dumbbells.

Sumo-Type Dead Lift With Barbell

Ab Strength (Back)
Slow

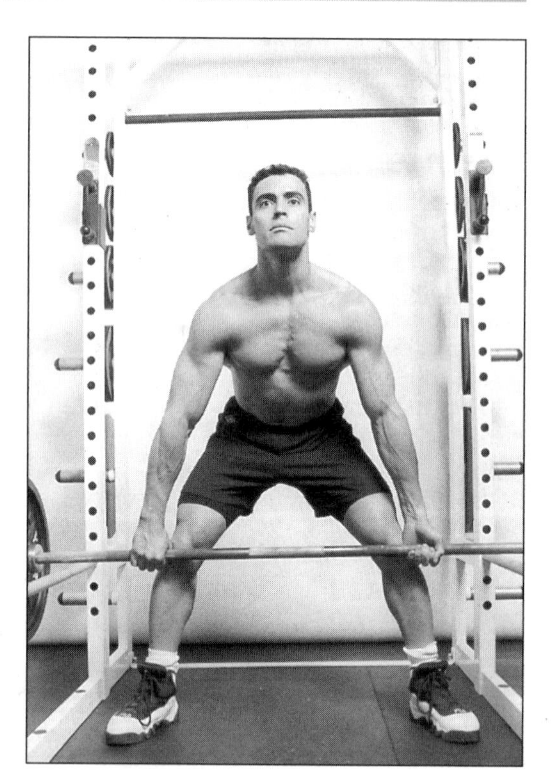

PREPARATION

- To begin, select a light weight, only increasing the resistance as strength level and mastery of technique dictate.
- Using a power rack, place the barbell at slightly lower than knee level.
- Place feet considerably wider than shoulder-width apart.
- Flex knees slightly.
- Bend at the waist.
- Grasp the bar outside of the knees.
- Use an over-under grip (one palm faces forward and the other faces back) to prevent the bar from rolling.
- Keep the back straight.
- Keep the head up.

ACTION

- Start the movement by lifting with the legs.
- Contract the low back muscles and gluteals, standing erect (do not hyperextend or arch the low back).
- Keep the back straight and the back musculature "tight" throughout the movement.
- Keep legs straight at the top of the movement.
- Keep arms straight and the bar close to the body.
- Slowly return to the starting position by first flexing at the knees, then the hips.
- Immediately repeat (do not bounce or jerk the bar to gain momentum).

Note: We advise caution for individuals with a history of low back pain or injury. Inhale up, exhale down. You can do this exercise using dumbbells.

Low Back or Hip and Back

Ab Strength (Back)
Slow to Moderate

PREPARATION

- Many machines will vary as to the mechanical design.
- Follow the guidelines suggested by the manufacturer.

ACTION

- Follow the manufacturer's directions for the exercise.

8

Ab Power Exercises

Physical training is one of the most neglected aspects of sports participation. Most programs devote an inordinate amount of time to the enhancement of sport-specific skills such as dribbling, passing, spiking, and slap shots, while little time is spent developing athletic skills. Ultimately, it is athleticism that determines the *level* at which you can perform sport-specific skills. Training for heightened athleticism is the preparation of psychological and physiological attributes necessary for intense performance. It implies a harmonious relationship between the mind and the body. Fun? No, but it's the most important factor that separates the champions from the benchwarmers.

SYNERGISTIC TRAINING

Power training is typically reserved for the serious athlete. Because of the dynamic nature of competitive sports, it is necessary to train the explosive power of the trunk and torso *synergistically*. We can define *synergy* as the whole product being greater than the sum of its parts. There is an infinite combination of core movements (flexing, extending, rotating, and so on), and the planes in which they are performed. For example, side-to-side bending is done in the frontal plane; twisting is done in the rotational plane; and forward and backward bending is in the sagittal plane. Individually, each of these primary plane movements represents a part of the total. Enhancing each part of the whole product is certainly a major component of the athlete's regimen; yet he must also incorporate movements on many planes, thereby integrating a large proportion of the core musculature.

FUNCTIONAL TRAINING

The inclusion of activities that involve the *entire* trunk and torso, not just isolated muscle groups, represents *functional* power development. Choose activities that incorporate movements similar to the dominant energy systems and movement patterns specific to your particular sport or position. For example, functional movements for the discus thrower involve primarily rotational activities, the sprinter, mainly flexing and extending, and so on. Adhering to the concept of specificity, the discus thrower's primary training focus should mainly involve drills and activities that include a rotational component. A sprinter, who has little use for such a rotational element, should place considerably less emphasis (if any) on such training. Most sports require movements within all planes, so it will be up to you to determine your specific needs and where to place the emphasis in your training.

The core region is comprised primarily of slow-twitch fibers. This suggests that it is capable of sustaining large workloads with a rapid recovery. Yet, while slow-twitch fibers predominate, fast-twitch fibers are also present. Certainly, the core region is capable of performing explosive actions. In addition, the explosive movements of the extremities either originate, are stabilized by, or transfer through the center of power. Thus, the core is the essential link in the performance of all power movements. As a result, power development in the core must incorporate action that is both explosive and similar to actual movements of the sport for which you are training. This will elicit the recruitment and development of the fast-twitch musculature and concentrate all involved muscles into usable, functional patterns.

POWER ACTIVITIES

The abdominal exercises in this chapter are power activities. Many, but not all, of the exercises are plyometrics. Some of the exercises, however, do not fall into the plyometric category because they do not feature the characteristic short range-of-motion pre-stretch followed by an explosive contraction. But because of the higher speeds representative of the drills in this chapter and the fact that you must use medicine balls, which are often associated with plyometric training, we have cautiously categorized this chapter as power-oriented. We'll use the term "power" in the general sense to identify those activities that call for a little more speed per repetition than did earlier exercises.

Training for power differs dramatically from strength and endurance training. If you will recall from chapter 1, a plyometric exercise is one that focuses on the neural aspects of muscle development. Four important physiological transformations occur as a result of plyometric training:

1. It enhances the amount of elastic energy the muscle is able to store.
2. It "teaches" working muscles to contract more forcefully through a greater percentage of fiber involvement.
3. It stimulates neural pathways to develop a more efficient sequence of motor unit firing, referred to as the "summation of forces."
4. It strengthens the impulses that inhibit the slowing effects of an unwanted simultaneous contraction of the antagonistic (opposing) muscles.

Plyometric training will help your muscles function more efficiently and therefore will enhance power output. In short, plyometrics train the speed component of power through neuromuscular avenues.

Guidelines for Power Activities

The following guidelines will help you determine if you are physically capable of safely performing the drills in this chapter:

1. If you are contemplating including these power-oriented drills in your existing training regimen, we can only assume that you are earnestly participating in athletics. These exercises have little use in the general population. Advancement on to this chapter indicates that you have the physical capacity to successfully perform the majority of the drills illustrated in the previous two chapters. Look over the ab strength training program we outline in chapter 9. If you are deemed not ready for its regimen, then you are definitely not ready to begin these drills.
2. Always warm up first. A vigorously exercised muscle that is inadequately prepared is vulnerable to injury. As you glance at the exercises outlined in this chapter, you will notice explosive, sometimes violent, tendencies. Most sports contain a similar ballistic component. It is dangerous to perform these exercises "cold." Therefore, we strongly suggest that you precede each training session with a complete and thorough warm-up, including both static flexibility and active movements. Be

sure to choose warm-up activities that closely mimic the movement patterns of the exercises you plan to do and gradually build velocity.

3. Determining the appropriate intensity is always a challenge. Remember that more is not always better. You should start at a level that represents your current conditioning status. The photographs in this chapter show the athlete using a 3-kilo (6.6-pound) medicine ball. But don't think that this is the minimal weight to reap the benefits of conditioning. Start low, master the technique, and progress slowly. You may want to start using a volleyball, then progress to a 1-kilo medicine ball, then to a 2-kilo, and so on. You may find that some exercises are more difficult than others. Therefore, you may not progress to the heavier weight balls as rapidly in some drills as in others.
4. Correct technique is critical. Never sacrifice technique to advance to a heavier resistance or add repetitions or sets. If you're not sure your technique is proper, have a training partner who is familiar with the technique assess your efficiency or watch yourself in a mirror to receive immediate feedback.
5. Because of the increased risk of injury, never perform power exercises when fatigued. While the number of repetitions per set may range from 10 to 25, the total number of repetitions per session will be low (under 300). Make sure to allow for significant rest (one minute minimum) between sets.

POWER EXERCISES

Standing Trunk Rotation With Arms Tight

Ab Power (Obliques)
Fast

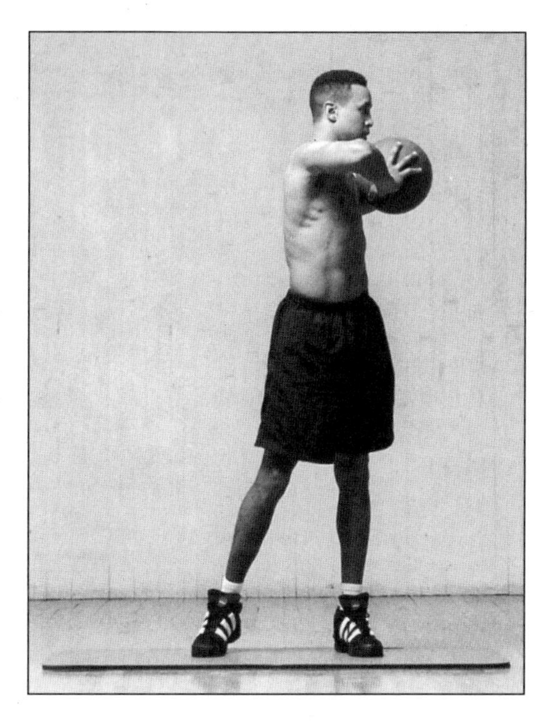

PREPARATION

- Stand tall.
- Place feet shoulder-width apart.
- Flex knees slightly.
- Lean weight slightly forward on the balls of the feet.
- Maintain a tight and controlled trunk and torso.
- Hold the ball to the chest, elbows flared out.
- To start, turn the shoulders and face left.

ACTION

- Contract the right obliques and quickly twist the upper body and ball to the right.
- Without pausing, immediately counter the momentum of the ball, snapping back to the left.
- Allow the feet to pivot. This will decrease the rotational stress on the knees.
- Immediately repeat.

Note: As you grow stronger, increase the weight of the ball. However, never sacrifice technique for added resistance.

Standing Trunk Rotation With Arms Extended

Ab Power (Obliques)
Fast

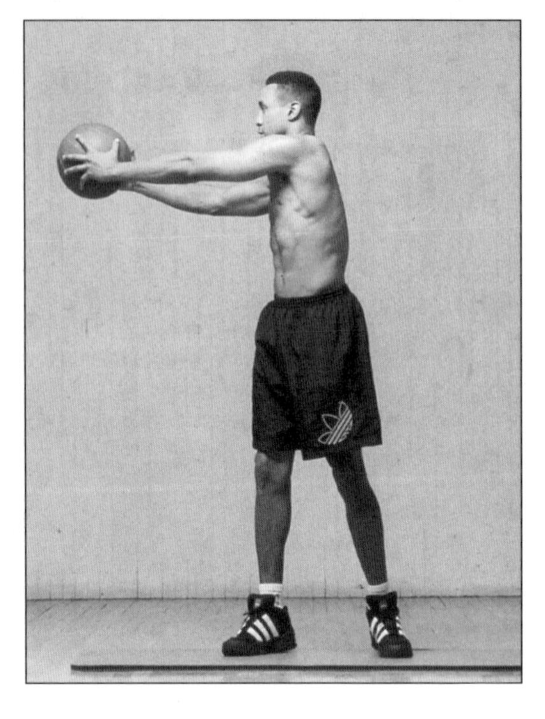

PREPARATION

- Stand tall.
- Place feet shoulder-width apart.
- Flex knees slightly.
- Lean weight slightly forward on the balls of the feet.
- Maintain a tight and controlled trunk and torso.
- Grasp the ball with arms extended at chest level.
- To start, turn the shoulders and face left.

ACTION

- Contract the right obliques and quickly twist the upper body and ball to the right.
- Without pausing, immediately counter the momentum of the ball, snapping back to the left.
- Allow the feet to pivot. This will decrease the rotational stress on the knees.
- Immediately repeat.

Note: As you grow stronger, increase the weight of the ball. However, never sacrifice technique for added resistance.

Seated Trunk Rotation With Arms Tight

Ab Power (Obliques)
Fast

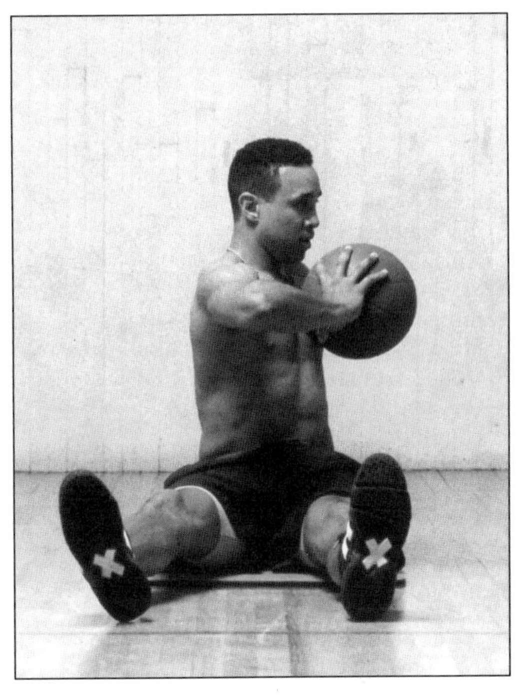

PREPARATION

- Sit on the floor with legs straight.
- Place feet at least shoulder-width apart.
- Sit tall.
- Keep head up.
- Maintain a tight and controlled trunk and torso.
- Hold the ball to the chest, elbows flared out.
- To start, turn shoulders and face left.

ACTION

- Contract the right obliques and quickly twist the upper body and ball to the right.
- Without pausing, immediately counter the momentum of the ball, snapping back to the left.
- Immediately repeat.

Note: As you grow stronger, increase the weight of the ball. However, never sacrifice technique for added resistance.

Seated Trunk Rotation With Arms Straight

Ab Power (Obliques)
Fast

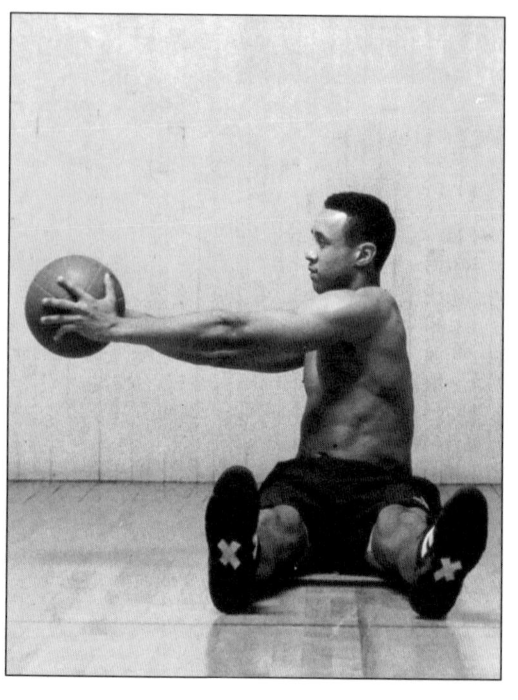

PREPARATION

- Sit on the floor with legs straight.
- Place feet at least shoulder-width apart.
- Sit tall.
- Keep head up.
- Maintain a tight and controlled trunk and torso.
- Grasp the ball with arms extended at chest level.
- To start, turn shoulders and face left.

ACTION

- Contract the right obliques and quickly twist the upper body and ball to the right.
- Without pausing, immediately counter the momentum of the ball, snapping back to the left.
- Immediately repeat.

Note: As you grow stronger, increase the weight of the ball. However, never sacrifice technique for added resistance.

Side Bend

Ab Power (Obliques)
Moderate

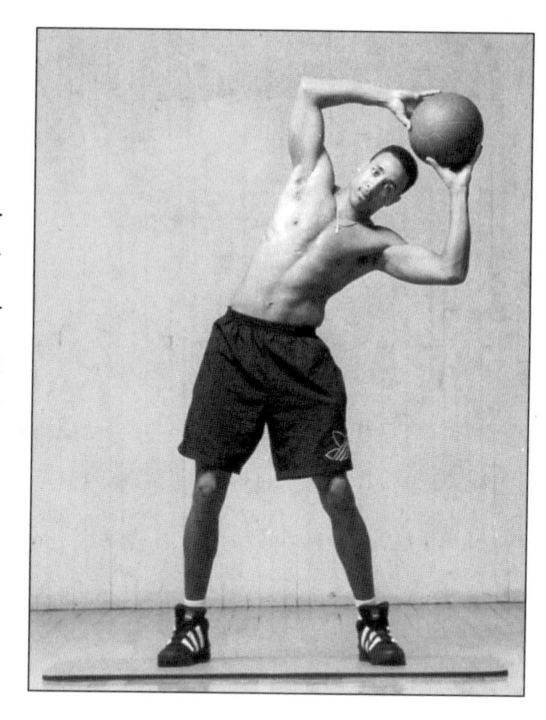

PREPARATION

- Stand tall.
- Place feet slightly wider than shoulder-width apart.
- Flex knees slightly.
- Maintain a tight and controlled trunk and torso.
- Hold the ball overhead close to, but not touching, the top of the head.

ACTION

- Bend to the left.
- Without stopping, immediately counter the momentum of the ball and bend to the right.
- Maintain erect upper body posture. Do not lean forward or backward.
- Immediately repeat.

Note: As you grow stronger, increase the weight of the ball. However, never sacrifice technique for added resistance.

Medicine Ball Russian Twist

Ab Power (Obliques)
Moderate

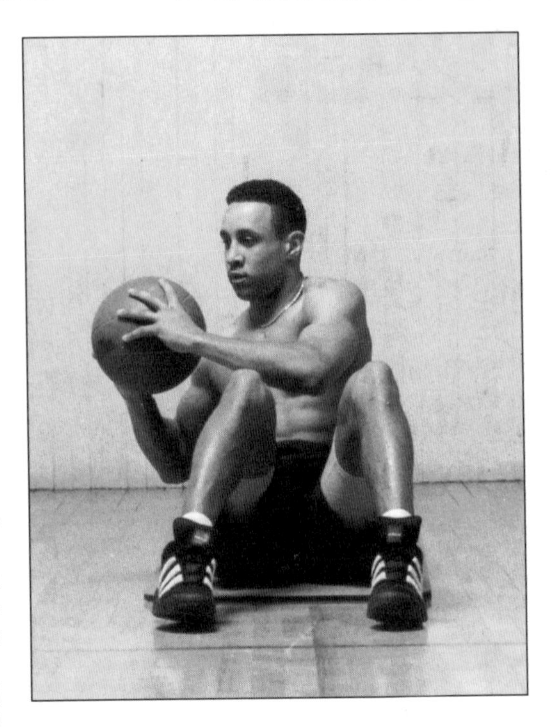

PREPARATION

- Lie on back.
- Place feet shoulder-width apart.
- Flex knees to 90 degrees.
- Grasp the ball.
- Flex elbows slightly.
- To start, hold the ball at shoulder level, face left, and tap the floor.

ACTION

- Contract the right obliques and upper abs.
- Twist to the right and lift the upper body approximately 45 degrees off the floor.
- Make the path of the ball pass over the knees and back down to the floor on the right side.
- Tap the floor on the right.
- Immediately repeat toward the opposite side.

Note: As you grow stronger, increase the weight of the ball. However, never sacrifice technique for added resistance.

Partner Side-to-Side Toss With Both Standing

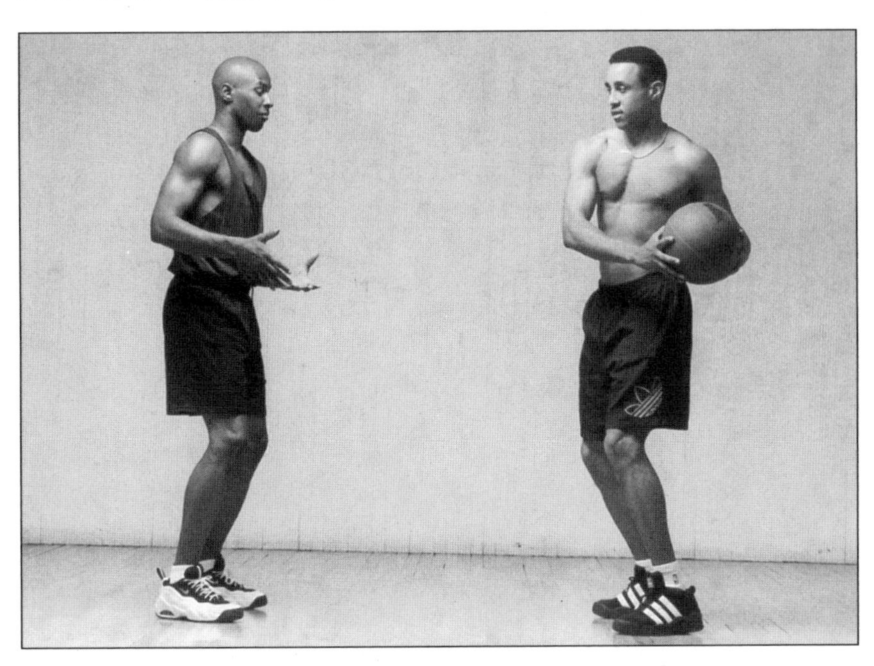

A B

Ab Power (Obliques)
Moderate

PREPARATION

- Partners stand facing each other, 5 to 10 feet apart.
- Stand tall.
- Place feet shoulder-width apart.
- Flex knees slightly.
- Maintain a tight and controlled trunk and torso.
- Athlete *B* holds ball at the side, waist high.
- To start, athlete *B* turns shoulders and faces left.

ACTION

- Athlete *B* tosses the ball from left hip to athlete *A*'s right hip (same side when facing).
- The momentum of the ball "forces" athlete *A* to twist to that side.
- Athlete *A* counters the momentum, immediately snapping the ball back to athlete *B*'s left side (same side as at beginning).
- Maintain correct posture.
- Do not lean forward or backward.
- Continue on the same side for one set.
- Repeat on the opposite side.

Note: As you grow stronger, increase the weight of the ball. However, never sacrifice technique for added resistance.

Partner-Assisted Rotation Toss With One Seated

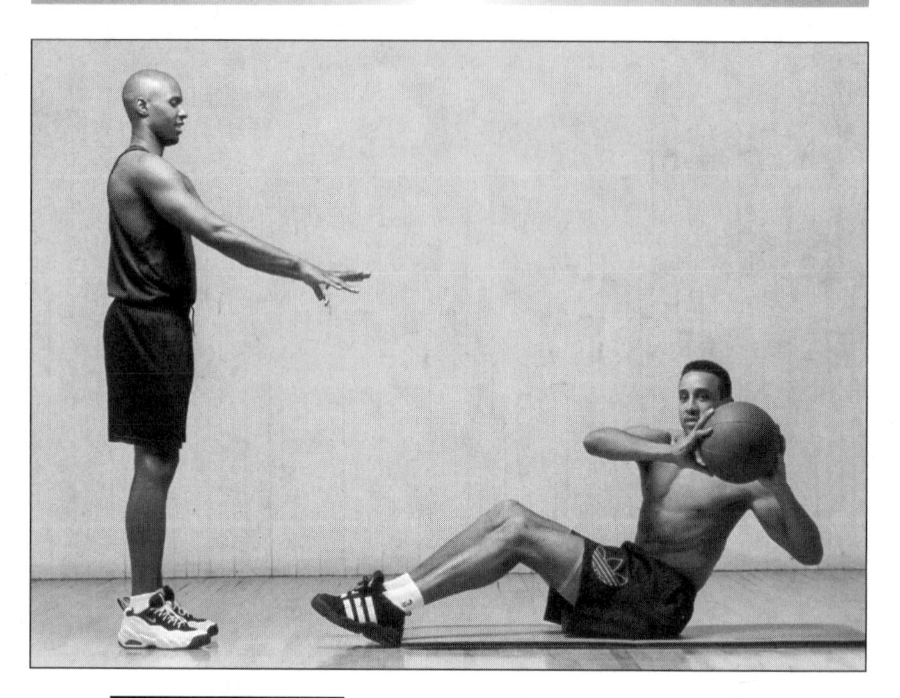

Ab Power (Obliques)
Moderate to Fast

PREPARATION

- The athlete who will be receiving the training sits, knees flexed to 90 degrees.
- Place feet shoulder-width apart.
- Sit tall.
- Hold hands at face level, ready to catch the ball.
- Focus eyes on the ball.
- The other athlete stands a comfortable distance away (from inches to several feet), holding the ball.

ACTION

- The athlete who is standing tosses the ball to the left side of the seated athlete. Throw the ball slightly *above* the left shoulder of the seated athlete. (At first, the toss should be soft; as strength and coordination improves, increase the velocity of the toss.)
- When the seated athlete catches the ball, the momentum drives him back toward the floor.
- Control the downward momentum, tapping the ball on the floor (do not bounce).
- The athlete quickly rises back to the starting position while simultaneously tossing the ball to the standing partner.
- Keep the ball over the shoulder and not in front of the body.
- Continue toward the same side for one set.
- Repeat toward the opposite side.

Note: As you grow stronger, increase the weight of the ball. However, never sacrifice technique for added resistance. If the seated athlete requires assistance to complete the movement, have the partner stand lightly on the seated athlete's feet.

Partner Cross Toss With Both Standing

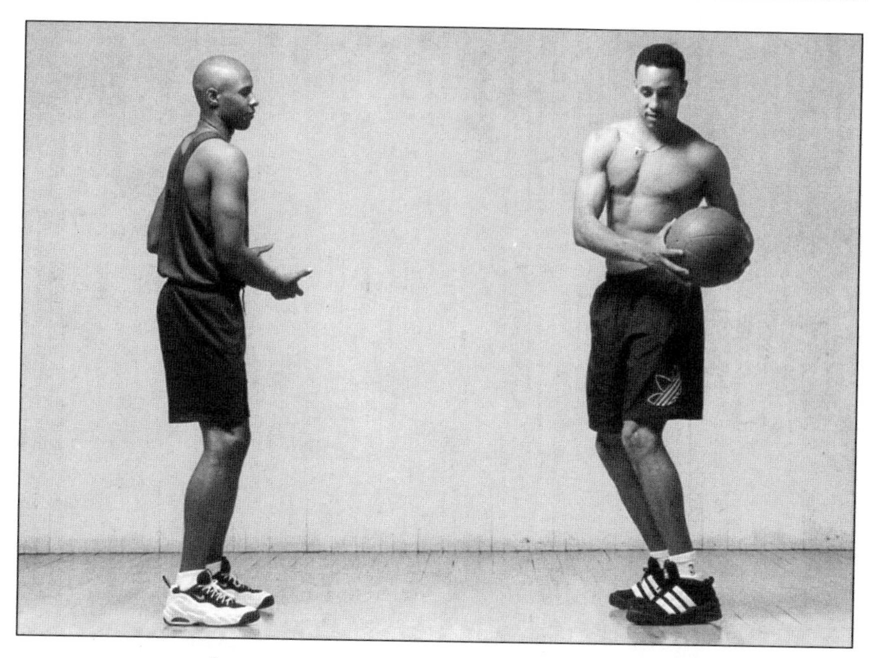

Ab Power (Obliques)
Fast to Explosive

PREPARATION

- Partners stand facing each other, 5 to 10 feet apart.
- Stand tall.
- Place feet shoulder-width apart.
- Flex knees slightly.
- Maintain a tight and controlled trunk and torso.
- Athlete *B* holds the ball at the side, waist high.
- To start, athlete *B* turns shoulders and faces left.

ACTION

- Athlete *B* tosses the ball diagonally across to the left side of athlete *A*.
- The momentum "forces" athlete *A* to twist to that side.
- Athlete *A* counters the momentum, immediately snapping the ball back across to athlete *B*'s left side (same side as at beginning).
- Maintain correct posture.
- Do not bend forward or backward.
- Continue left-side tosses for one set.
- Repeat toward the opposite side.

Note: As you grow stronger, increase the weight of the ball. However, never sacrifice technique for added resistance.

Partner Cross Toss With Both Seated

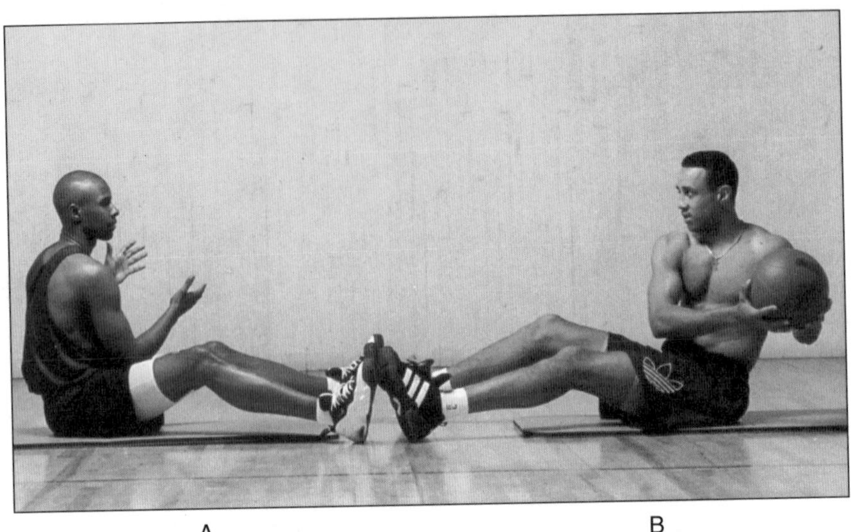

A B

Ab Power (Obliques)
Moderate to Fast

PREPARATION

- Both athletes sit on the floor facing each other, a comfortable distance apart.
- Place feet shoulder-width apart.
- Flex knees slightly.
- Sit tall.
- Hold hands up, ready to receive the ball.
- Focus eyes on the ball.
- Athlete *B* holds the ball waist high.
- To start, athlete *B* turns shoulders and faces left.

ACTION

- Athlete *B* tosses the ball diagonally across to the left side of athlete *A*.
- The momentum will "force" athlete *A* to twist to that side.
- Athlete *A* counters the momentum, immediately snapping the ball back across to athlete *B*'s left side (same side as at beginning).
- Maintain correct posture.
- Do not lean forward or backward.
- Continue left-side tosses for one set.
- Repeat toward the opposite side.

Note: As you grow stronger, increase the weight of the ball. However, never sacrifice technique for added resistance.

Standing Wall Cross Toss

Ab Power (Obliques)
Explosive

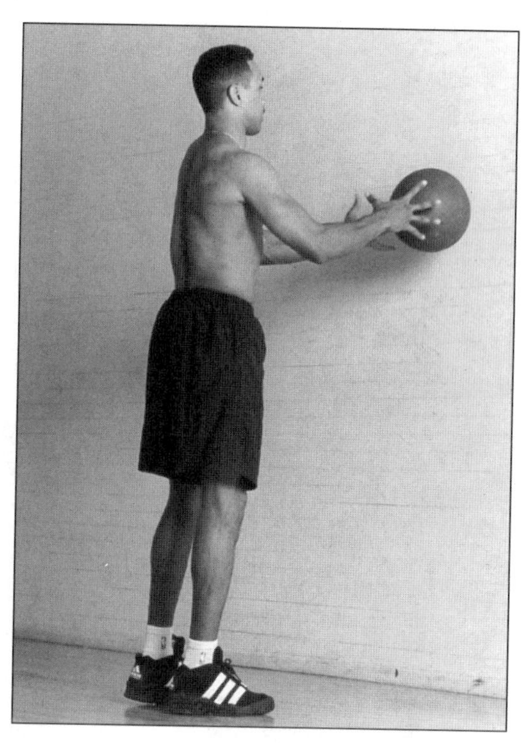

PREPARATION

- Stand tall, facing a *solid* wall, four to six feet away.
- Place feet shoulder-width apart.
- Flex knees slightly.
- Maintain a tight and controlled trunk and torso.
- Flex elbows slightly.
- Hold ball slightly above waist level.
- To start, turn shoulders and face left.

ACTION

- Snap the hips (low torso) and toss the ball diagonally to the wall.
- Direct the ball so it will contact the wall higher than the released position.

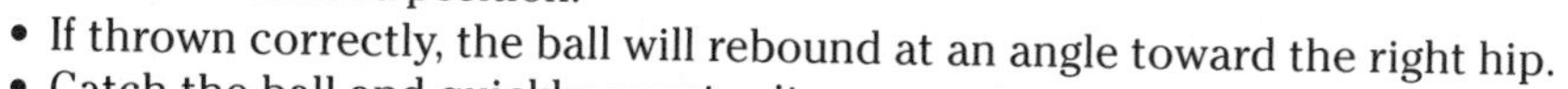

- If thrown correctly, the ball will rebound at an angle toward the right hip.
- Catch the ball and quickly counter its momentum.
- Snap the hips (low torso) back toward the wall.
- Do not throw the ball with the arms or upper body; instead, focus on explosive oblique action.
- Continue, alternating sides for one set.

Note: As you grow stronger, increase the weight of the ball. However, never sacrifice technique for added resistance.

Seated Wall Cross Toss

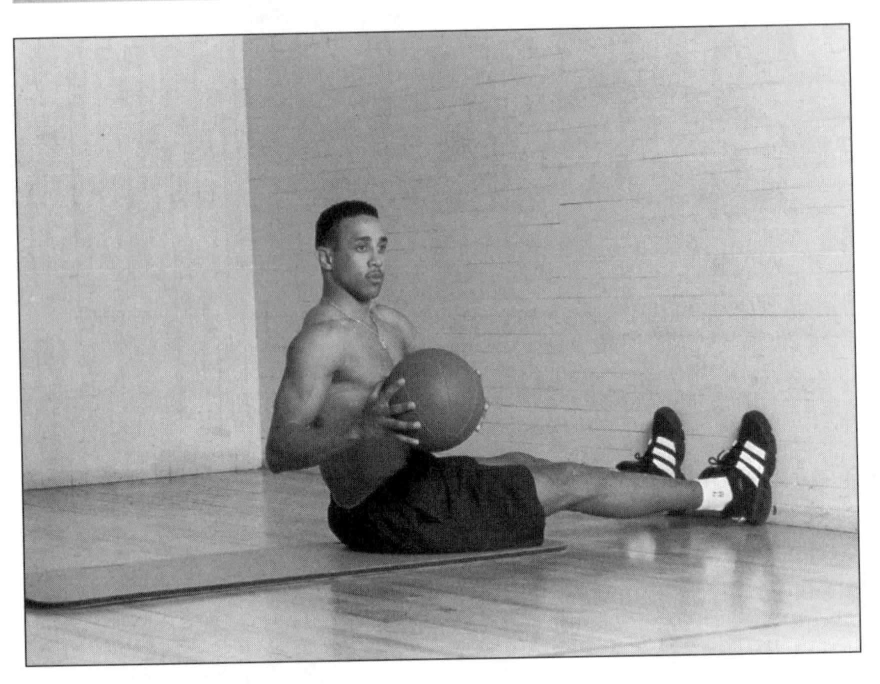

Ab Power (Obliques)
Explosive

PREPARATION

- Sit facing a *solid* wall.
- Spread legs slightly wider than shoulder-width apart.
- Touch wall with feet. (As strength and coordination improve, move farther away from the wall.)
- Sit tall.
- Maintain a tight and controlled trunk and torso.
- Flex elbows slightly.
- Hold ball slightly above waist level.
- To start, turn shoulders and face left.

ACTION

- Snap the hips (low torso) and toss the ball diagonally to the wall.
- Direct the ball so it will contact the wall higher than the released position.
- If thrown correctly, the ball will rebound at an angle toward the right hip.
- Catch the ball and quickly counter its momentum.
- Snap the hips (low torso) back toward the wall.
- Do not throw the ball with the arms or upper body; instead, focus on explosive oblique action.
- Continue, alternating sides for one set.

Note: As you grow stronger, increase the weight of the ball. However, never sacrifice technique for added resistance.

Standing Partners Reverse Twist Handoff

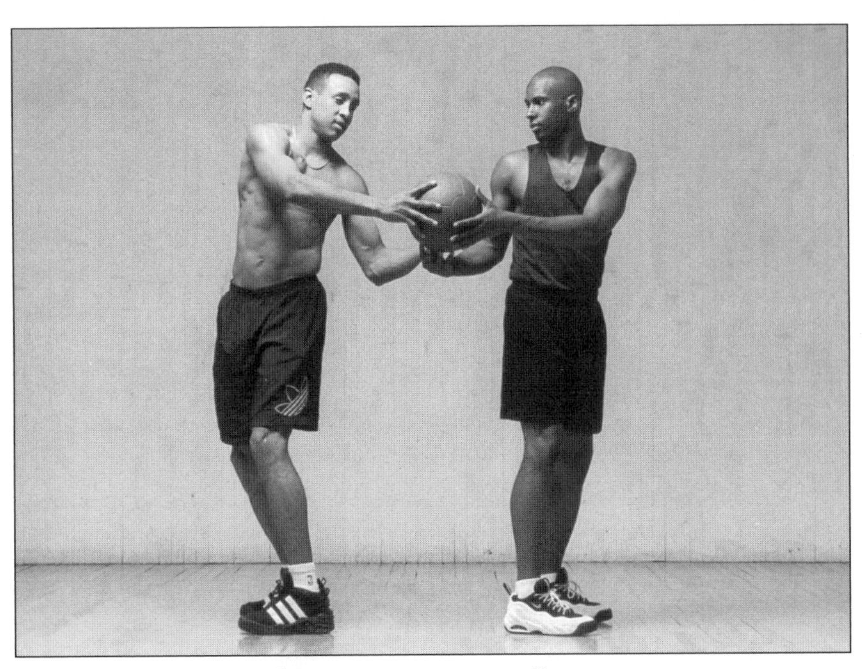

A B

Ab Power (Obliques)
Fast to Explosive

PREPARATION

- With a partner, stand tall, back-to-back, approximately two arm's-lengths apart.
- Place feet shoulder-width apart.
- Flex knees slightly.
- Maintain a tight and controlled trunk and torso.
- Hold arms parallel to the floor.
- Flex elbows slightly.

ACTION

- Athlete *A* holds the ball away from the body and twists to the left.
- Athlete *B* positions to receive the handoff on the right side.
- Athlete *B* immediately twists to the left and *hands* the ball off to athlete *A*'s right side (do not *toss* the ball).
- Allow the feet to pivot, decreasing the rotational stress on the knees.
- Continue toward the same direction for one set.
- Repeat toward the opposite direction.

Note: As you grow stronger, increase the weight of the ball. However, never sacrifice technique for added resistance.

Seated Partners Reverse Twist Handoff

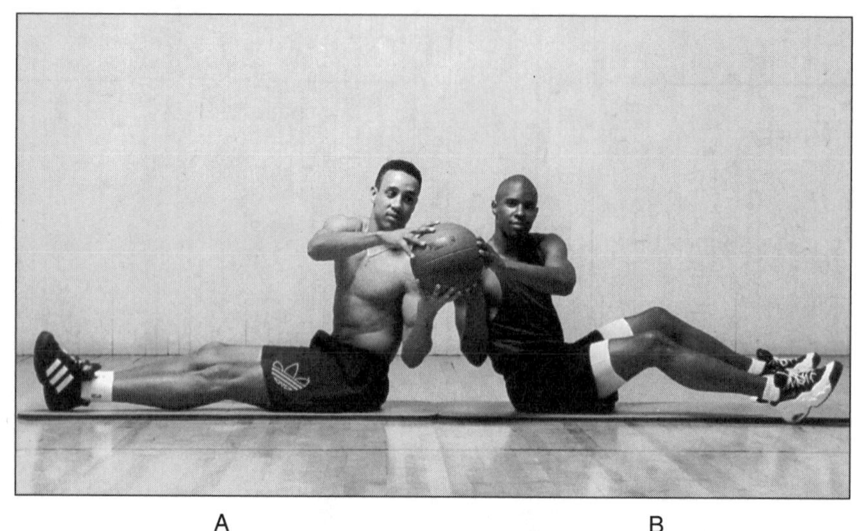

A B

Ab Power (Obliques)
Fast to Explosive

PREPARATION

- Partners sit back-to-back on the floor, approximately two arm's-lengths apart.
- Spread legs.
- Flex knees slightly.
- Sit tall.
- Maintain a tight and controlled trunk and torso.
- Hold arms parallel to the floor.
- Flex elbows slightly.

ACTION

- Athlete *A* holds the ball away from the body and twists to the left.
- Athlete *B* positions to receive the handoff on the right side.
- Athlete *B* immediately twists to the left and hands the ball off to athlete *A*'s right side (do not *toss* the ball).
- Continue toward the same direction for one set.
- Repeat toward the opposite direction.

Note: As you grow stronger, increase the weight of the ball. However, never sacrifice technique for added resistance.

Standing Partners Reverse Twist Toss

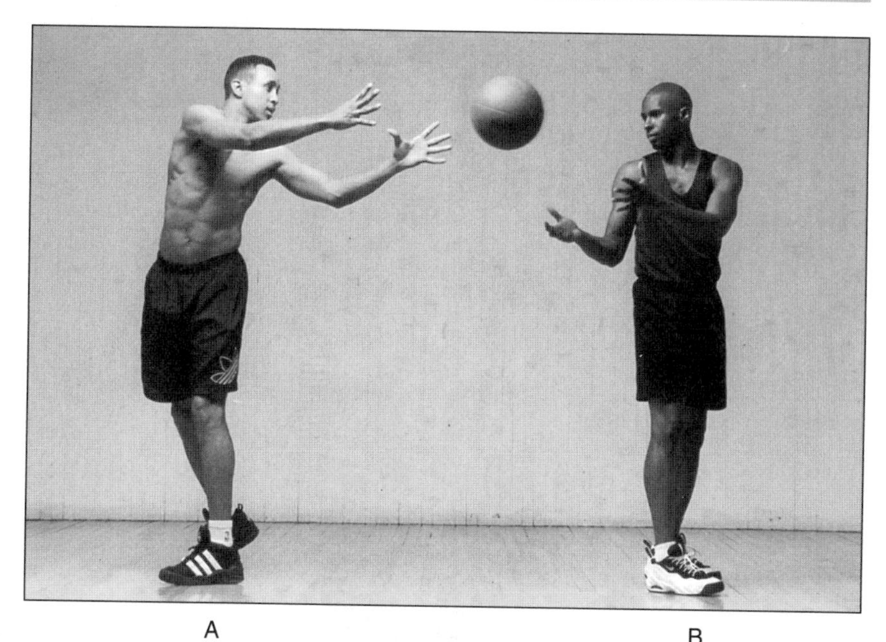

Ab Power (Obliques)
Explosive

PREPARATION

- Partners stand tall, back-to-back.
- Distance apart will vary, depending on the strength levels of the athletes and experience with the exercise. To begin, try five feet.
- Place feet shoulder-width apart.
- Flex knees slightly.
- Lean weight slightly forward on the balls of the feet.
- Maintain a tight and controlled trunk and torso.
- Hold arms parallel to the floor.
- Flex elbows slightly.

ACTION

- Athlete *A* holds the ball away from the body and twists to the left, *tossing* the ball to athlete *B*.
- Athlete *B* positions to catch the ball on the right.
- Athlete *B* immediately twists to the left and *tosses* the ball back to athlete *A*'s right side.
- Do not throw the ball with the arms; instead, focus on explosive oblique action.
- Allow the feet to pivot, decreasing the rotational stress on the knees.
- Continue toward the same direction for one set.
- Repeat toward the opposite direction.

Note: As you grow stronger, increase the weight of the ball. However, never sacrifice technique for added resistance.

Seated Partners Reverse Twist Toss

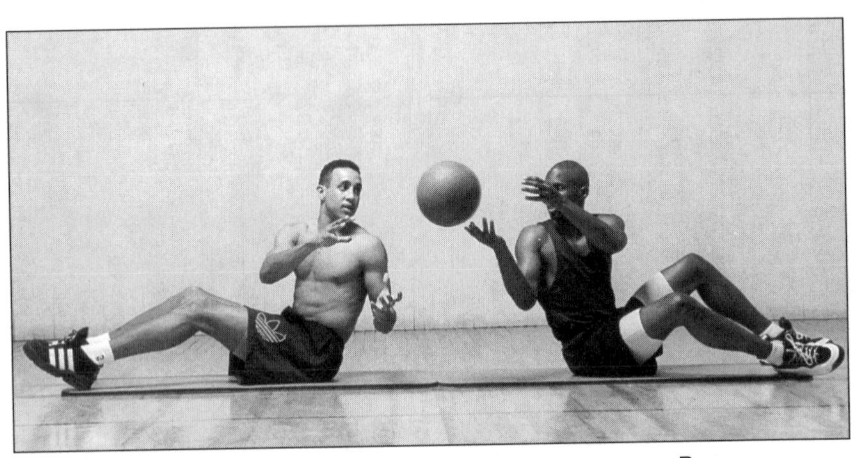

A B

Ab Power (Obliques)
Explosive

PREPARATION

- Partners sit back-to-back on the floor.
- Distance apart will vary, depending on the strength levels of the athletes and their experience with the exercise. To begin, try five feet.
- Spread legs.
- Flex knees slightly.
- Sit tall.
- Maintain a tight and controlled trunk and torso.
- Hold arms parallel to the floor.
- Flex elbows slightly.

ACTION

- Athlete *A* holds the ball away from the body and twists to the left tossing the ball to athlete *B*.
- Athlete *B* positions to catch the ball on the right side.
- Athlete *B* immediately twists to the left and *tosses* the ball back to athlete *A*'s right side.
- Do not throw the ball with the arms; instead, focus on explosive oblique action.
- Continue toward the same direction for one set.
- Repeat toward the opposite direction.

Note: As you grow stronger, increase the weight of the ball. However, never sacrifice technique for added resistance.

Standing Partners Medicine Ball Snap Handoff

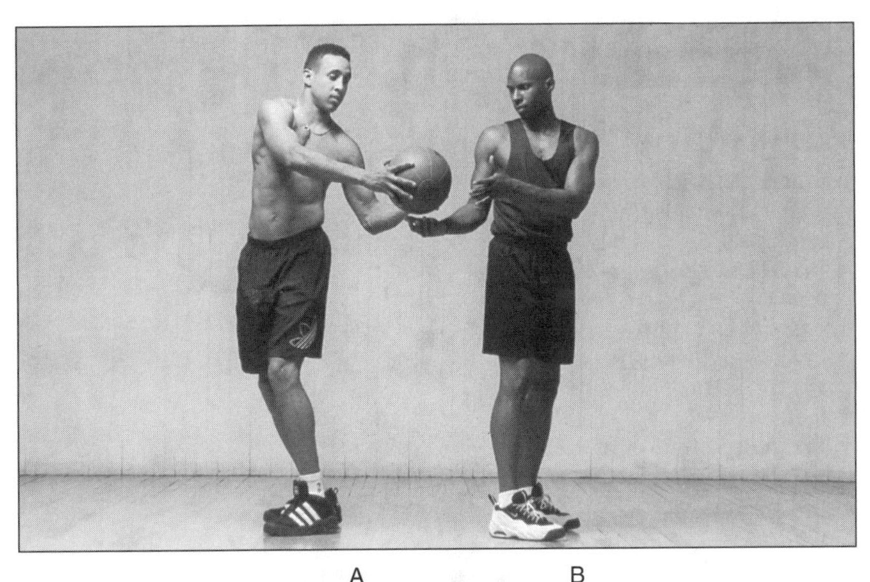

Ab Power (Obliques)
Explosive

PREPARATION

- Partners stand tall, back-to-back, approximately two arm's-lengths apart.
- Place feet shoulder-width apart.
- Flex knees slightly.
- Lean weight slightly forward on the balls of the feet.
- Maintain a tight and controlled trunk and torso.
- Hold arms parallel to the floor.
- Flex elbows slightly.

ACTION

- Athlete *A* holds the ball away from the body and snaps the hips to the left.
- Athlete *B* positions to receive the ball on the right side.
- Athlete *A hands* the ball to athlete *B*.
- Athlete *B* stops the ball's momentum at the mid-rotation point (i.e., arms straight ahead), keeping the elbows slightly flexed.
- Athlete *B* immediately snaps the hips back to the right and hands the ball off to athlete *A*'s left side.
- Allow the feet to pivot, decreasing the rotational stress on the knees.
- Continue toward the same direction for one set.
- Repeat toward the opposite side.

Note: As you grow stronger, increase the weight of the ball. However, never sacrifice technique for added resistance.

Medicine Ball Snap Toss to a Wall

Ab Power (Obliques)
Explosive

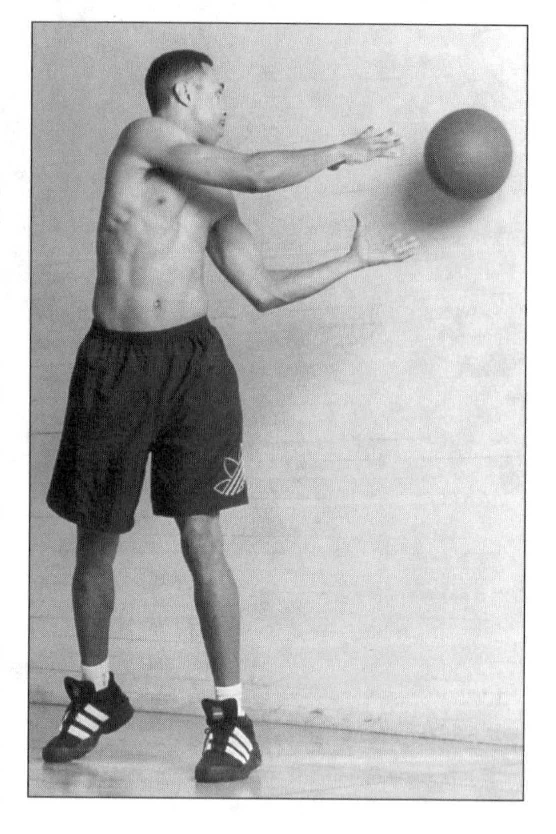

PREPARATION

- Stand tall with back to a *solid* wall that is four to six feet away.
- Place feet shoulder-width apart.
- Flex knees slightly.
- Lean weight slightly forward on the balls of the feet.
- Maintain a tight and controlled trunk and torso.
- Hold arms parallel to the floor.
- Flex elbows slightly.

ACTION

- Snap the hips (low torso) to the left and *toss* the ball to the wall.
- Direct the ball so that it contacts the wall and rebounds back to the same side.
- Catch the ball and stop its momentum at the mid-rotation point (i.e., arms straight ahead), keeping elbows slightly flexed.
- Immediately snap the hips in the direction opposite the momentum, tossing the ball back to the wall on the left side.
- Allow the feet to pivot, decreasing the rotational stress on the knees.
- Continue toward the same side for one set.
- Repeat toward the opposite side.

Note: As you grow stronger, increase the weight of the ball. However, never sacrifice technique for added resistance.

Freestanding Knee-Ups

Ab Power (Lower)
Moderate to Fast

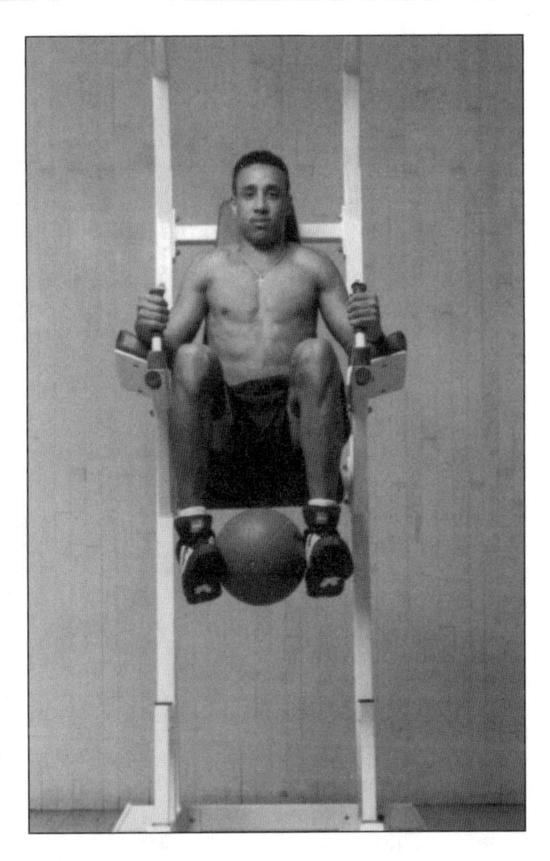

PREPARATION

- Position lumbar support pad properly to provide support for the low back.
- Position elbows on the elbow support pads, aligned with or slightly in front of the upper body.
- Firmly grip the handles.
- Extend legs toward the floor.
- Grasp the ball between the ankles.

ACTION

- Lift the ball, quickly bringing the knees toward the chest.
- Hold for one count (i.e., "one-thousand-one").
- Slowly return to the starting position. Do not swing; instead, control the ball movement.
- Immediately repeat.

Note: Start with a very light ball or no ball at all. As you grow stronger, increase the weight of the ball. However, never sacrifice technique for added resistance. We advise the use of a training partner to assist you, ensuring correct technique.

Hanging Knee-Ups

Ab Power (Lower)
Moderate

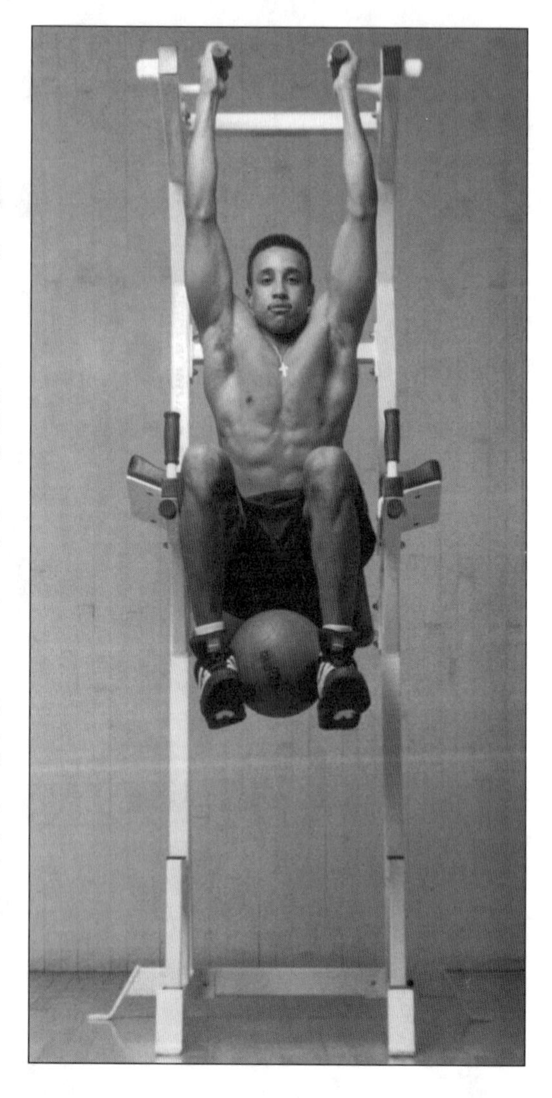

PREPARATION

- Hang from an overhead bar, arms fully extended.
- Grasp the ball between the ankles.

ACTION

- Lift the ball, quickly bringing the knees toward the chest. Do not swing and avoid pulling up with the arms.
- Maintain a slight hunch in the back. Do not hyperextend the low back.
- Slowly return to the starting position.
- Immediately repeat.

Note: Start with a very light ball or no ball at all. As you grow stronger, increase the weight of the ball. However, never sacrifice technique for added resistance. We advise the use of a training partner to assist you, ensuring correct technique. Use wrist straps or elbow slings if shoulder and arm strength is inadequate to facilitate correct technique.

Roman Chair Crunch

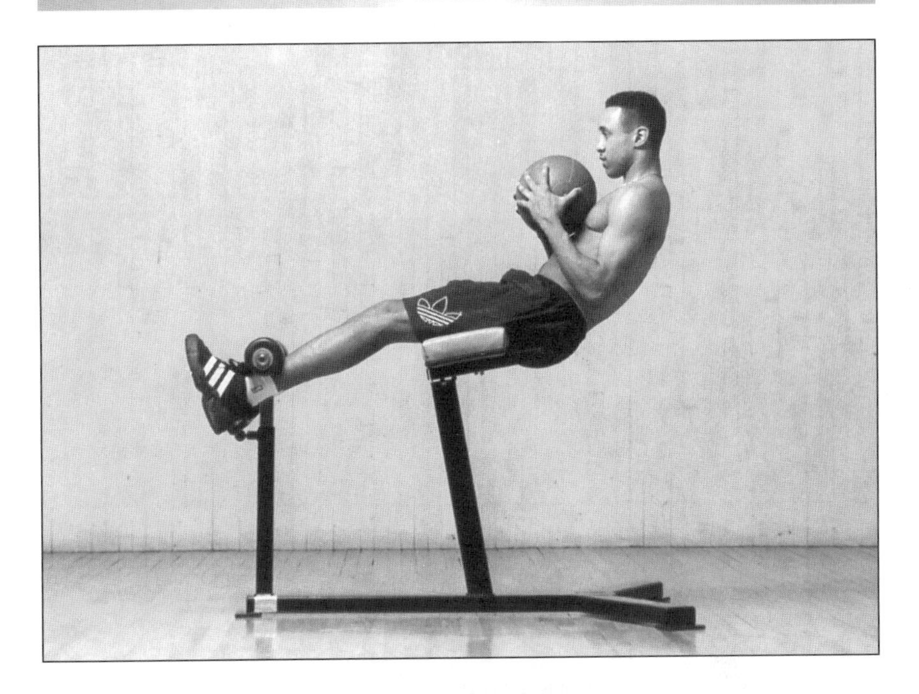

Ab Power (Upper)
Slow to Moderate

Warning: This must be a very controlled exercise; do not perform during a state of extreme fatigue, risking improper technique.

PREPARATION

- Sit upright on the Roman Chair with the tibia (lower leg) pads properly adjusted.
- Position hips on the front edge of the torso pad.
- Hold the ball tightly to the chest.

ACTION

- Lower the upper body back to a position almost parallel to the ground.
- Rise to a position approximately 45 degrees above parallel.
- Slowly return to the starting position and repeat. Do not hyperextend the low back.

Note: Keep a slight "roll" to the spine. This will help eliminate hyperextension of the low back. As you grow stronger, increase the weight of the ball. However, never sacrifice technique for added resistance. Also, as strength level improves, position the ball farther away from the point of axis. For example, if strength level is low, start with the ball at the waist and, as strength level improves, move the ball to the chest and, finally, above the head.

Beginning Medicine Ball Crunch

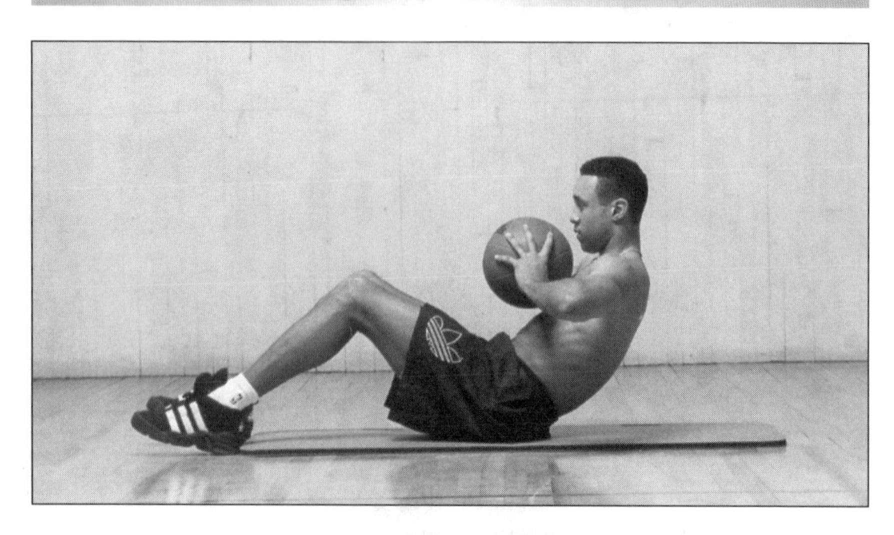

Ab Power (Upper)
Moderate

PREPARATION

- Lie on the floor on the back.
- Place feet shoulder-width apart.
- Flex knees to 90 degrees. (If strength level is low, you may want to hook your feet under a heavy object for added leverage.)
- Hold the ball to the chest.

ACTION

- Quickly raise the upper body to approximately 45 degrees to the floor.
- Slowly lower the upper body to the floor.
- Tuck chin to the chest, keeping a slight "roll" in the spine to help eliminate hyperextension of the low back.
- Tap the shoulder blades (do not bounce).
- Immediately repeat.

Note: As you grow stronger, increase the weight of the ball. However, never sacrifice technique for added resistance.

Advanced Medicine Ball Crunch

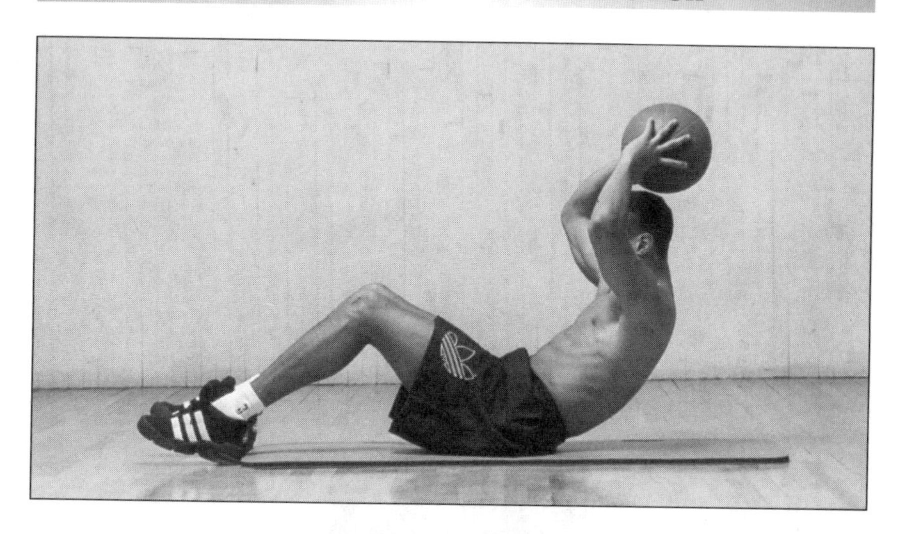

Ab Power (Upper)
Moderate

PREPARATION

- Lie on the floor on the back.
- Place feet shoulder-width apart.
- Flex knees to 90 degrees. (If strength level is low, you may want to hook your feet under a heavy object for added leverage.)
- Hold the ball close to, but not touching, the head.

ACTION

- Raise the upper body approximately 45 degrees to the floor.
- Keep the ball directly overhead.
- Slowly lower the upper body to the floor.
- Tuck chin to the chest, keeping a slight "roll" in the spine to help eliminate hyperextension of the low back.
- Tap the shoulder blades (do not bounce) and immediately repeat.

Note: As you grow stronger, increase the weight of the ball. However, never sacrifice technique for added resistance.

One-Seated Partner-Assisted Chest Pass Crunch

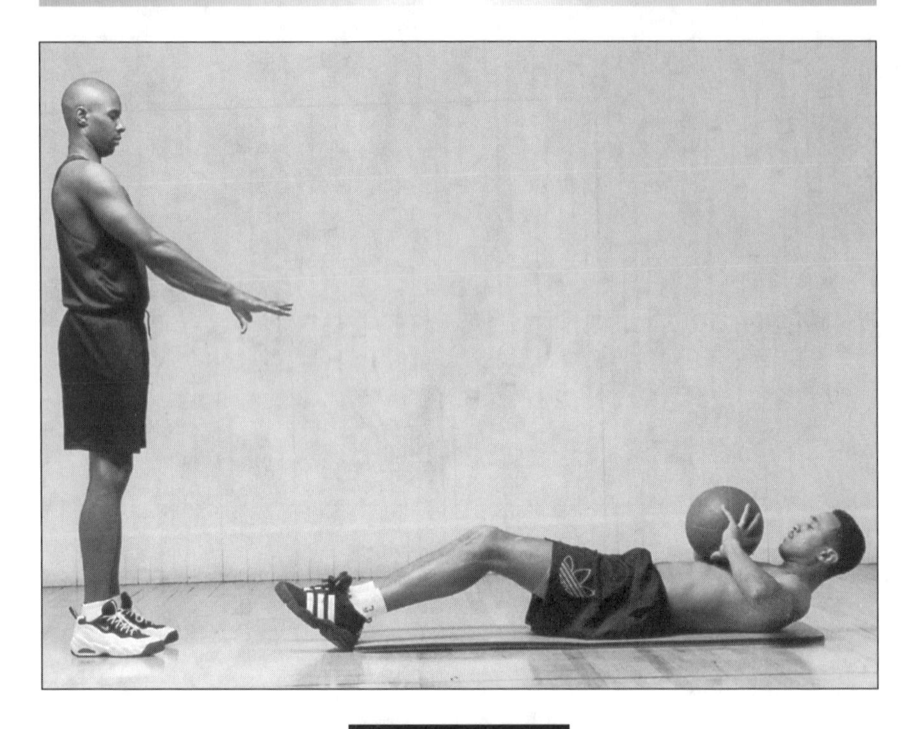

Ab Power (Upper)
Fast

PREPARATION

- The athlete who will be receiving the training sits with knees flexed to 90 degrees.
- Place feet shoulder-width apart.
- Sit tall.
- Hold hands up at chest level, ready to receive the ball.
- Focus eyes on the ball.

ACTION

- The athlete who is standing tosses the ball to the chest of the seated athlete. (To begin, the toss should be soft; as strength and coordination improve, increase the velocity of the toss.)
- When the ball is caught, the momentum will drive the seated athlete back toward the floor.
- Control the downward momentum and tap the shoulder blades to the floor (do not bounce).
- Tuck chin to the chest, keeping a slight "roll" in the spine to help eliminate hyperextension of the low back.
- The seated athlete quickly rises back to the starting position while simultaneously tossing the ball to the standing partner.
- Immediately repeat.

Note: As you grow stronger, increase the weight of the ball. However, never sacrifice technique for added resistance. If the seated athlete requires assistance to complete the movement, have the partner stand lightly on the seated athlete's feet.

One-Seated Partner-Assisted Overhead Throw Crunch

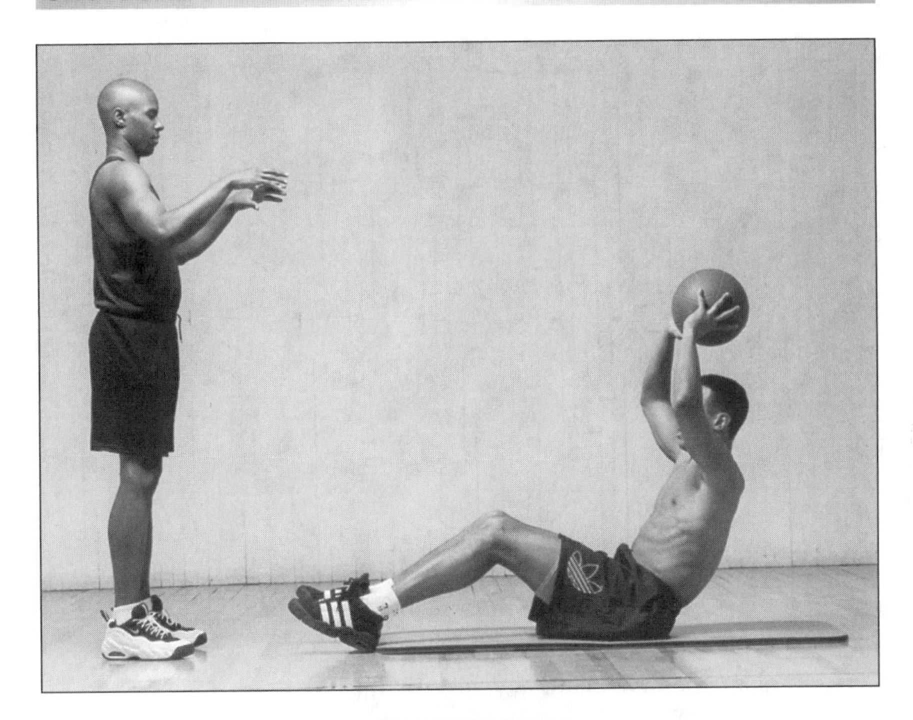

Ab Power (Upper)
Moderate

PREPARATION

- The athlete who will be receiving the training sits with knees flexed to 90 degrees.
- Place feet shoulder-width apart.
- Sit tall.
- Hold hands above the head, ready to receive the ball.
- Focus eyes on the ball.

ACTION

- The athlete who is standing tosses the ball to the waiting hands of the seated athlete. (To begin, the toss should be soft; as strength and coordination improve, increase the velocity of the toss.)
- When the ball is caught, the momentum will drive the seated athlete back toward the floor.
- Control the downward momentum and tap the ball to the floor (do not bounce).
- Tuck chin to the chest, keeping a slight "roll" in the spine to help eliminate hyperextension of the low back.
- Keep the ball overhead at all times.
- The seated athlete quickly rises back to the starting position while simultaneously tossing the ball back to the standing partner.
- Immediately repeat.

Note: As you grow stronger, increase the weight of the ball. However, never sacrifice technique for added resistance. If the seated athlete requires assistance to complete the movement, have the partner stand lightly on the seated athlete's feet.

Seated Partners Chest Pass Crunch

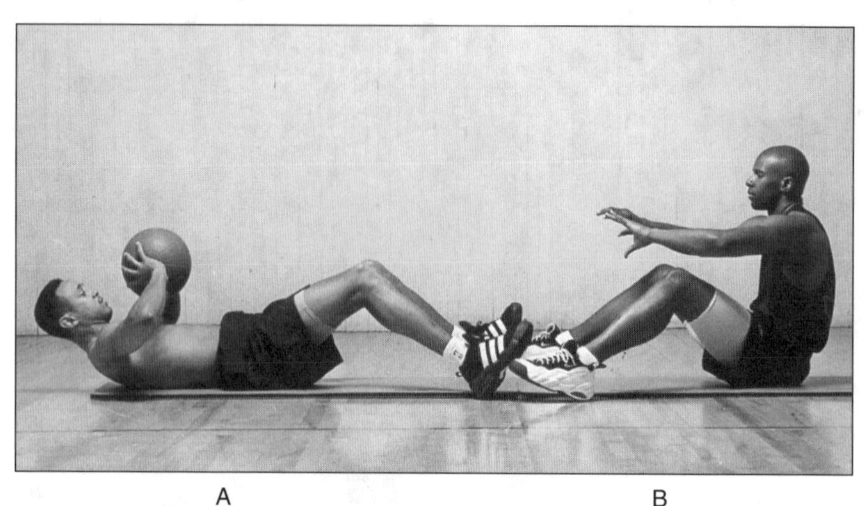

A B

Ab Power (Upper)
Fast

PREPARATION

- Both athletes sit on the floor facing each other.
- Place feet shoulder-width apart.
- Flex knees slightly.
- Sit tall.
- Athlete *B*'s hands are at chest level, ready to receive the ball.
- Flare elbows out.
- Focus eyes on the ball.
- Athlete *A* holds ball at chest level.

ACTION

- Athlete *A* throws a chest pass to athlete *B*.
- When the ball is caught, the momentum will drive athlete *B* back toward the floor.
- Athlete *B* controls the downward momentum and taps the shoulder blades to the floor (do not bounce).
- Tuck chin to the chest, keeping a slight "roll" in the spine to help eliminate hyperextension of the low back.
- Athlete *B* quickly rises up to the starting position while simultaneously tossing the ball to the chest of athlete *A*.
- Maintain correct posture.
- Continue for one set.

Note: As you grow stronger, increase the weight of the ball. However, never sacrifice technique for added resistance. For added leverage, athlete *A* hooks the right ankle under athlete *B*'s left, and athlete *B* hooks the right ankle under athlete *A*'s left.

Seated Partners Overhead Toss Crunch

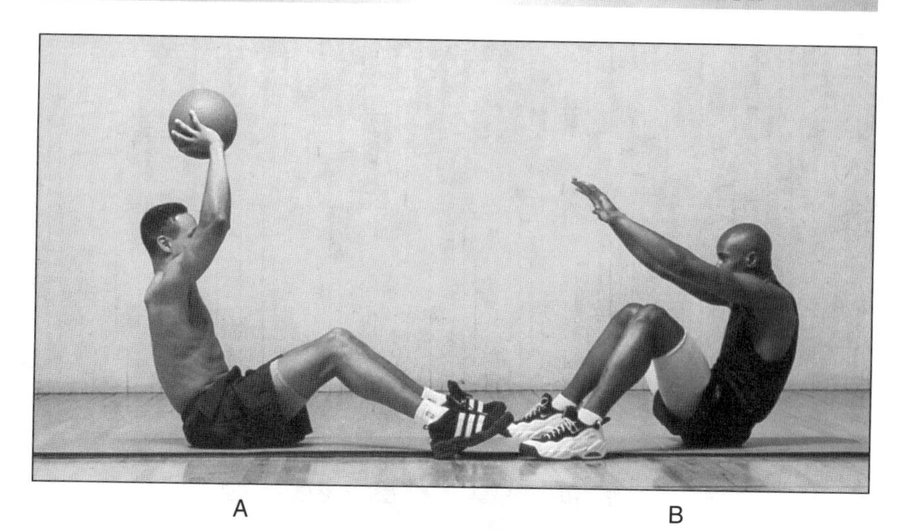

A B

Ab Power (Upper)
Fast

PREPARATION

- Both athletes sit on the floor facing each other.
- Place feet shoulder-width apart.
- Flex knees slightly.
- Sit tall.
- Hold hands above the head, ready to receive the ball.
- Flex elbows slightly.
- Focus eyes on the ball.

ACTION

- Athlete *A* tosses the ball overhead to the waiting hands of athlete *B*.
- When the ball is caught, the momentum will drive athlete *B* back toward the floor.
- Athlete *B* controls the downward momentum and taps the ball to the floor (do not bounce).
- Tuck chin to the chest, keeping a slight "roll" in the spine to help eliminate hyperextension of the low back.
- Athlete *B* quickly rises up to the starting position while simultaneously tossing the ball overhead to athlete *A*.
- Maintain correct posture.
- Continue for one set.

Note: As you grow stronger, increase the weight of the ball. However, never sacrifice technique for added resistance. For added leverage, athlete *A* hooks the right ankle under athlete *B*'s left, and athlete *B* hooks the right ankle under athlete *A*'s left.

Wall Chest Pass

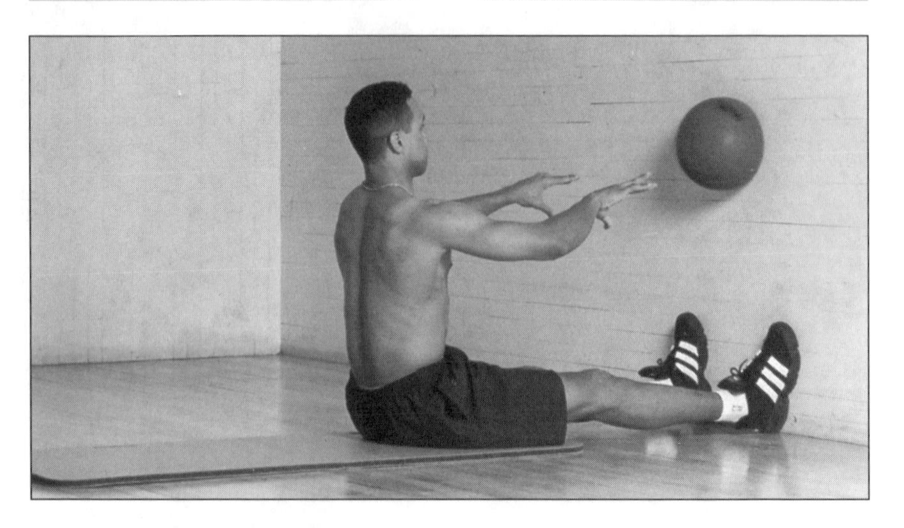

Ab Power (Upper)
Fast

PREPARATION

- Sit facing a *solid* wall.
- Spread legs slightly wider than shoulder-width apart.
- Touch the wall with the feet. (As strength and coordination improve, move farther away from the wall.)
- Sit tall.
- Maintain a tight and controlled trunk and torso.
- Hold ball at chest level.
- Flare elbows out.

ACTION

- To start, toss the ball against the wall high enough so that you can catch the rebound at chest level.
- When you catch the ball, the momentum will drive you back toward the floor.
- Control the downward momentum and tap the shoulder blades to the floor (do not bounce).
- Tuck chin to the chest, keeping a slight "roll" in the spine to help eliminate hyperextension of the low back.
- Quickly rise to the starting position while simultaneously tossing the ball back to the wall.
- Catch the rebound.
- Immediately repeat.

Note: As you grow stronger, increase the weight of the ball. However, never sacrifice technique for added resistance. A variation of this exercise involves a limited range of motion. Rather than tapping the shoulder blades to the floor, "check" the downward momentum and stop the upper body at approximately 45 degrees to the floor.

Overhead Wall Toss

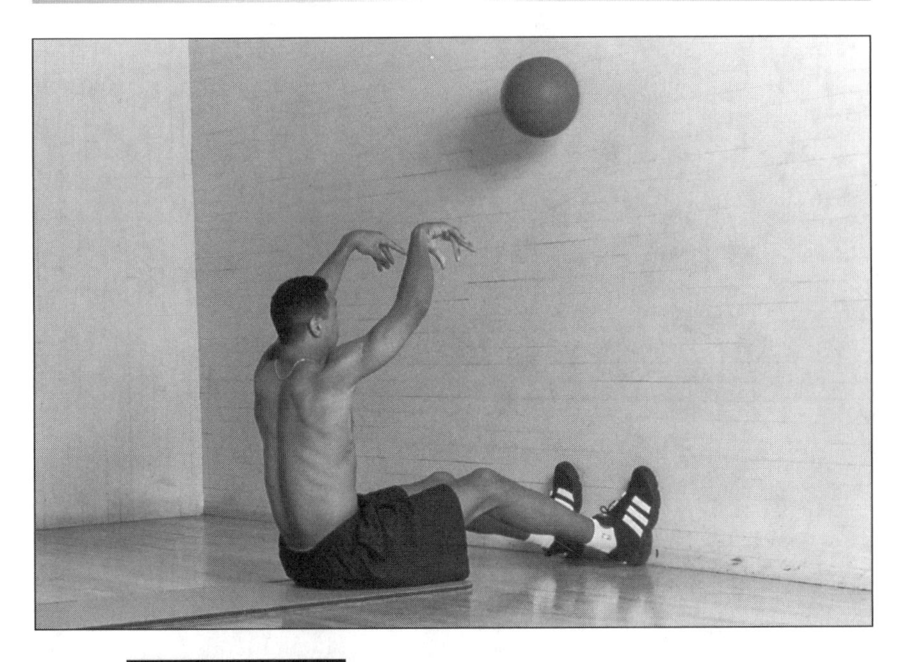

Ab Power (Upper)
Fast

PREPARATION

- Sit facing a *solid* wall.
- Spread legs slightly wider than shoulder-width apart.
- Touch the wall with the feet. (As strength and coordination improve, move farther away from the wall.)
- Sit tall.
- Maintain a tight and controlled trunk and torso.
- Hold the ball with arms extended overhead.
- Flex elbows slightly.

ACTION

- To start, toss the ball against the wall high enough so that you can catch the rebound above the head.
- When you catch the ball, the momentum will drive you back toward the floor.
- Control the downward momentum and tap the ball to the floor (do not bounce).
- Tuck chin to the chest, keeping a slight "roll" in the spine to help eliminate hyperextension of the low back.
- Quickly rise to the starting position while simultaneously tossing the ball back to the wall.
- Throw the ball with the abdominals, not the arms.
- Keep the ball overhead at all times.
- Catch the rebound.
- Immediately repeat.

Note: As you grow stronger, increase the weight of the ball. However, never sacrifice technique for added resistance. A variation of this exercise involves a limited range of motion. Rather than tapping the ball to the floor, "check" the downward momentum and stop the upper body at approximately 45 degrees to the floor.

Medicine Ball Back Crunch

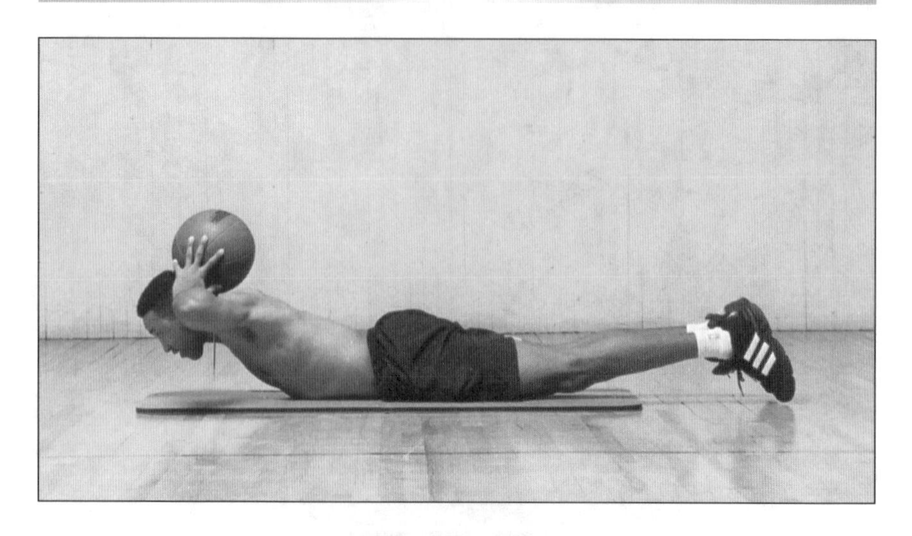

Ab Power (Back)
Slow to Moderate

PREPARATION

- Lie on the floor on the stomach.
- Hold the ball behind the head.

ACTION

- Contract the low back muscles and gluteals and raise the upper body off the floor.
- Hold the arched position for several counts.
- Slowly return to the starting position.
- Immediately repeat.

Note: Start with a very light ball or no ball at all. As you grow stronger, increase the weight of the ball. A variation of this exercise involves a lift with a twist.

Roman Chair Back Extension

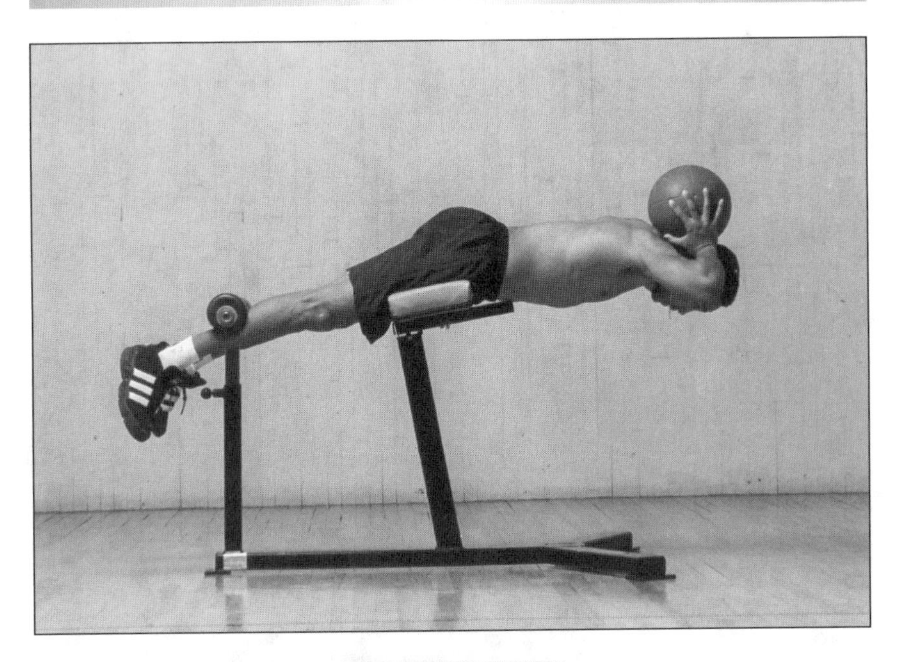

Ab Power (Back)
Slow to Moderate

Warning: This must be a very controlled exercise; do not perform during a state of extreme fatigue, risking improper technique.

PREPARATION

- Lie on the stomach on the Roman Chair with the ankle supports (tibia pads) properly adjusted and the hips on the support pads.
- Place the ball behind the head.

ACTION

- To start, hips are flexed, pointing head toward the floor.
- Contract the low back muscles and gluteals and raise the upper body to a position parallel to the floor.
- Slowly return to the starting position. (Do not bounce.)
- Immediately repeat.

Note: Start with a very light ball or no ball at all. As you grow stronger, increase the weight of the ball. A variation of this exercise involves a lift with a twist.

Medicine Ball Good Mornings

Ab Power (Back)
Slow

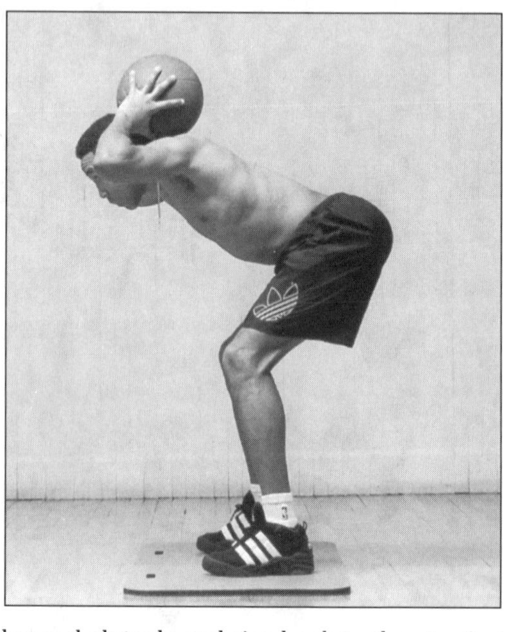

PREPARATION

- Stand tall.
- Place feet shoulder-width apart.
- Flex knees slightly.
- Maintain a tight and controlled trunk and torso.
- Start with the ball at waist level. As you grow stronger, move the ball to the chest and, eventually, behind the head.

ACTION

- Slowly lean forward until the upper body is almost parallel to the floor.
- Contract the low back muscles and gluteals and rise back to the starting position.
- Do not hyperextend the low back.
- Immediately repeat.

Note: Start with a very light ball or no ball at all. As you grow stronger, increase the weight of the ball.

Back Toss

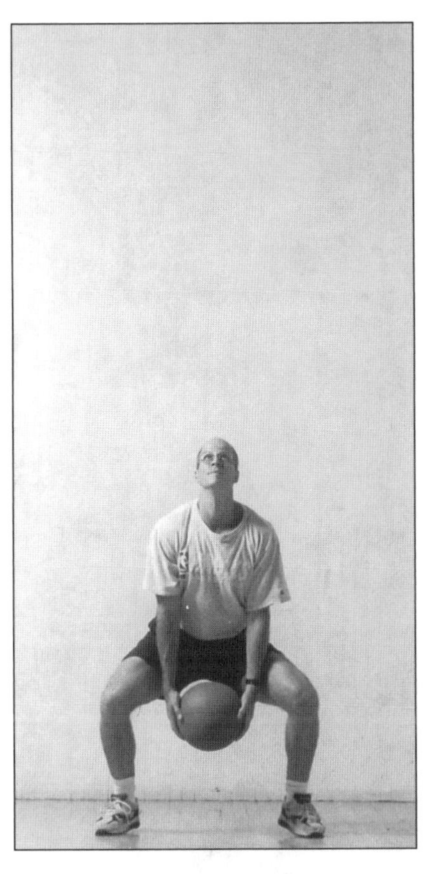

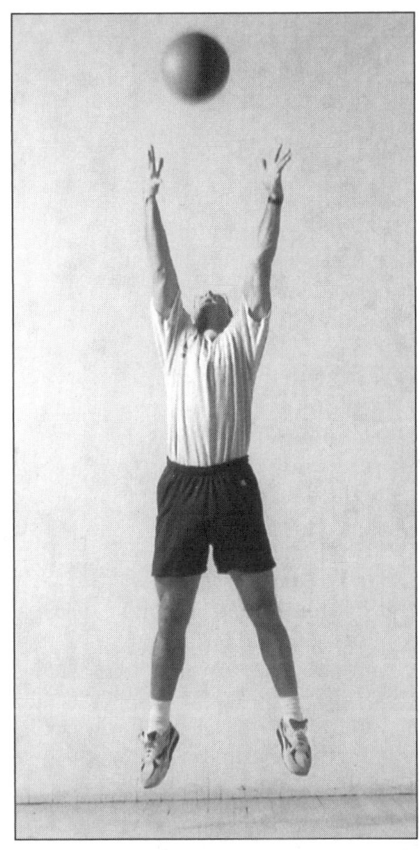

Ab Power (Back)
Explosive

PREPARATION

- Stand tall.
- Place feet shoulder-width apart.
- Extend arms downward with elbows slightly flexed.
- Hold ball at waist level.

ACTION

- Simultaneously squat and initiate a slight swing of the ball down and between the legs.
- "Drive" the legs up while lifting with the low back.
- Throw the ball as high as possible, making sure it lands behind you.
- *Always* watch the ball! Be careful the ball does not drop down on your head.
- This is an explosive movement—you should leave the ground during the throw.
- Retrieve the ball.
- Repeat.

Note: Avoid extreme hyperextension of the low back. As you grow stronger, increase the weight of the ball. However, never sacrifice technique for added resistance.

9

Abs and Back Training Program

Now it is time to bring together everything you've learned about ab and back fitness, strength, and power and to apply it to your own training. Begin with the ab fitness program and work your way up to level X. You may choose to remain at this level indefinitely if you have achieved your fitness goals, but if you want to progress beyond fitness to conditioning that will translate to higher-level performance as an athlete, go on to the ab strength program. Once you are securely established at the fitness and strength levels, you can consider progressing to the ab power program only if you are involved in serious athletics. For safety reasons, only elite-level athletes should attempt the ab power program and even these individuals should approach the program intelligently and with caution.

AB FITNESS

The ab fitness program on page 227 is a 24-week program that will firm, shape, and tone your abdominals. It does not involve any external resistance such as weights. This program will serve as the foundation for the strength and power levels, or it may be the only program you ever need to use. It is recommended that you continue to include exercises from level X (with decreased frequency and/or duration) once you have completed the 24-week program, whether or not you plan to move on to ab strength and ab power conditioning.

At the bottom of page 227 is an example of what a typical routine might look like. For this example, we have chosen level IV. Remember: Since you have many more than the 12 exercises found in this routine to choose from, the individual exercises in your unique program may be quite different from those in this sample.

Abs and Back Training Precautions

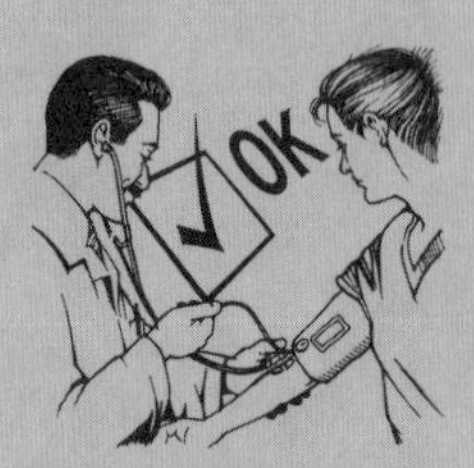

Get your doctor's approval before starting any new program.

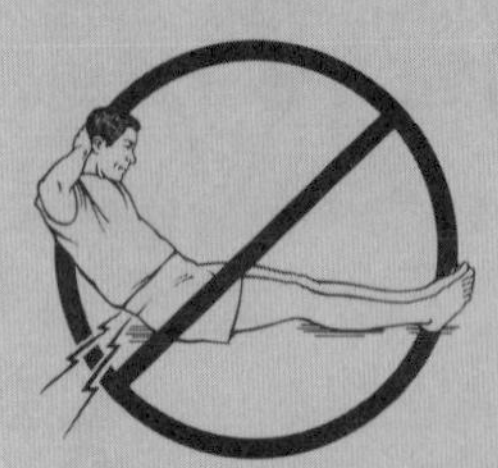

Avoid bilateral (double leg) straight leg lifts, straight-leg sit-ups, certain Roman Chair exercises, or any exercise that arches or severely hyperextends the low back. Always maintain low back support.

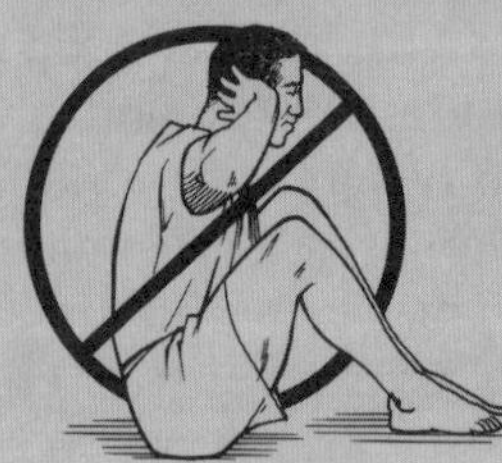

Conversely, avoid extreme flexing of the spine (specifically the low back).

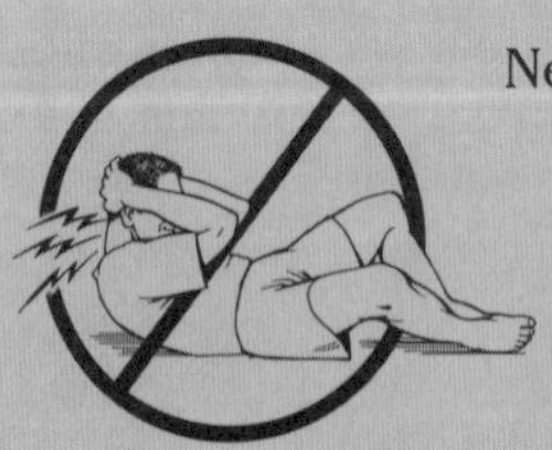

Never pull on the head or neck.

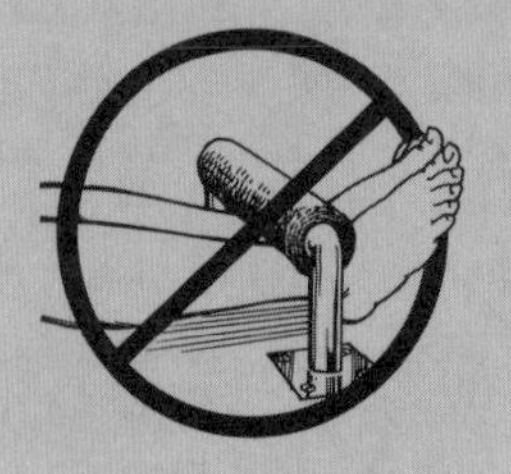

Avoid anchoring the feet unless there is no other way to successfully perform the lift.

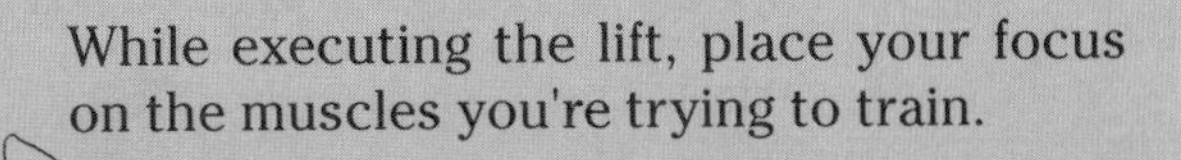

While executing the lift, place your focus on the muscles you're trying to train.

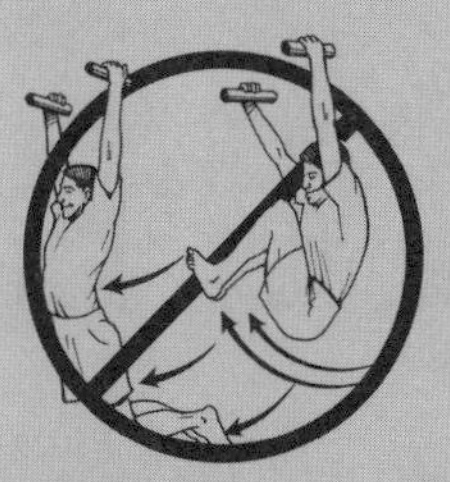

Avoid using jerking motions and momentum to accomplish the lift.

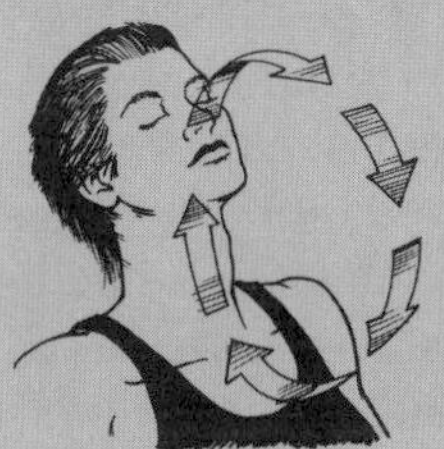

Breathe naturally and rhythmically.

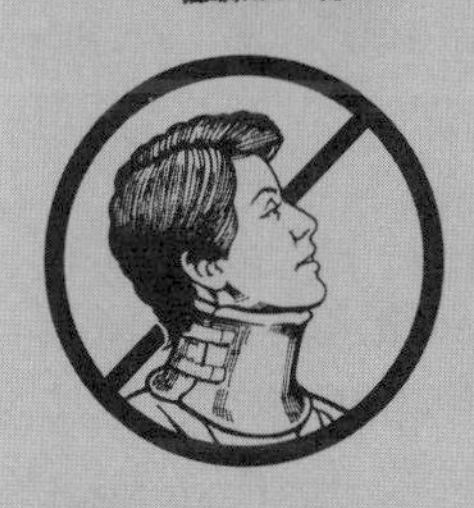

Never train while injured.

Ab Fitness Guidelines

- Always warm up prior to and cool down following any training session.
- Train all regions of the abdominals and low back, emphasizing imbalances.
- Choose 6 to 15 exercises that are marked "ab fitness" in their black boxes (chapter 6).
- Oblique exercises work both sides of the body and therefore count as two exercises.
- Initially, perform the routine four to five days per week. Avoid having several recovery days in a row. Space each training session evenly throughout the week. Upon reaching level X, keep intensity high; that is, maintain the level of difficulty as indicated by added resistance (arm and leg positions) or varying the speed of the exercise, but you can cut back the duration by eliminating *some* repetitions and sets and decrease frequency to two to four days per week if you wish. Remember, if you are satisfied with your progress at a lower level, by all means stay there. Advancement to subsequent levels does not necessarily mean continued or dramatic improvement. You may be perfectly content and adequately rewarded staying at a lower level forever.
- Never advance to the next level without first being able to accomplish the prescribed number of repetitions and sets while maintaining correct technique at your current level.
- Total abdominal repetitions during an ab fitness training regimen should not exceed 450 per session. (*Note:* This number does not include the back exercises.)
- Be sure to include low back exercises—20 to 100 total repetitions. For the ab fitness level, choose one to five back exercises (or more if this is an area you wish to concentrate on) and perform 5 to 20 repetitions.
- Upon reaching level IV, the beginning of multiple sets, perform all repetitions of each exercise, then rest one to two minutes before beginning subsequent sets.
- Rest between sets only. Do not rest between exercises.

24-Week Ab Fitness Program

Choose 6 to 15 exercises per session.

Level	Weeks	Repetitions per exercise	Sets per session
Initial Phase	4	4-6	1
I	2	8	1
II	2	10	1
III	2	12	1
IV	2	8	2
V	2	10	2
VI	2	12	2
VII	2	8	3
VIII	2	10	3
IX	2	12	3
X	2	15	3

Note: Continue at level X to *maintain* core fitness.

Ab Fitness Sample Daily Routine for Level IV: 2 Weeks

	Ab Fitness Exercises	Sets*	Repetitions
1.	Straight-Leg Side Crunch (Left)	2	8
2.	Straight-Leg Side Crunch (Right)	2	8
3.	Bent-Knee Side Raise (Left)	2	8
4.	Bent-Knee Side Raise (Right)	2	8
5.	Advanced Crossed-Leg Oblique Crunch (Left)	2	8
6.	Advanced Crossed-Leg Oblique Crunch (Right)	2	8
7.	Roll Back Isolate	2	8
8.	Seated Straight-Leg Tuck	2	8
9.	Butterfly Curl-Up	2	8
10.	Toes to Ceiling	2	8
11.	Russian Twist (Left)	2	8
12.	Russian Twist (Right)	2	8

*Perform one set of all twelve exercises, rest one minute, and repeat.
Total repetitions per session: 192

	Back Fitness Exercises	Sets	Repetitions
1.	Back Crunch	3	10
2.	Superman	3	10

AB STRENGTH

The ab strength routine is for individuals who are involved in competitive sports or who are more serious about their fitness training. You will notice that, unlike the 24-week ab fitness schedule, we do not structure an incremental routine for the following ab strength section. This is because we assume you have established a solid strength foundation through the successful completion of the level X ab fitness regimen.

AB STRENGTH GUIDELINES

- Always warm up prior to and cool down following any training session.
- Decrease frequency of ab fitness level X to two to three days per week but continue intensity and duration, keeping fitness repetitions to no more than 450 per session. *Note:* This is not a maintenance program, therefore you will not decrease intensity and duration (i.e., repetitions and sets).
- Incorporate ab strength exercises from chapter 7, two to three days per week.
- During ab strength training sessions, you may choose exercises from both ab fitness (chapter 6) and ab strength (chapter 7); however, emphasize ab strength exercises.
- Choose one to five exercises marked "ab strength" or "ab fitness."
- Oblique exercises work both sides of the body and therefore count as two exercises.
- Perform one to five sets of each exercise, 10 to 25 repetitions per set.
- Total abdominal repetitions during an ab strength training session should not exceed 350, though it is certainly not necessary to complete this many each and every session in order to receive training benefits. Because of the intensity or resistance used, time constraints, and equipment availability, your ab strength routine may not reach this maximum.
- Take a 30- to 120-second rest between *each set*, keeping it under 60 seconds if possible.

- Be sure to include low back exercises—20 to 100 total repetitions. For the ab strength level, choose one to five back exercises (or more if this is an area you wish to concentrate on). Do low back exercises marked "ab fitness" or "ab strength" and perform one to five sets of 5 to 20 repetitions.
- Remember, because of safety concerns, only elite-level athletes should move on to the ab power routine.

Ab Strength Sample Daily Routine

- **Maintain ab fitness level X, two to three days per week.**
- **Incorporate ab strength exercises from chapter 7 two to three other days per week.**

Ab Strength Exercises	Sets*	Repetitions
1. Flat Bench Oblique Crunch (Left)	2	15
2. Flat Bench Oblique Crunch (Right)	2	15
3. Freestanding Leg Raise—Bent-Knee	3	15
4. Seated Pull-Down Crunch	3	25
5. Roman Chair Upper Ab Isolate	1	25

*Rest approximately one minute between each set.
Total repetitions per session: 205

Back Strength Exercises	Sets	Repetitions
1. Roman Chair Back Crunch	3	10-15
2. Bent-Knee Dead Lift With Barbell	3	10

Note. Most athletes are involved in a comprehensive total body strength training routine that may already include several exercises that focus on low back development. If this is so, performing these low back exercises in conjunction with an abdominal routine would not be necessary.

AB POWER

We recommend the ab power routine for well-conditioned athletes *only*. You will design your own program based on the guidelines spelled out on page 230. Again, maintain your ab fitness and strength as discussed. Then gradually start incorporating ab power exercises but follow our guidelines carefully.

Ab Power Guidelines

- Always warm up prior to and cool down following any training session.
- Maintain ab fitness level X, two to three days per week, keeping fitness repetitions per session to 450 or less.
- Maintain ab strength one to two days per week.
- Incorporate ab power exercises from chapter 8, one to two days per week.
- Total ab training including all three levels should be four to six days per week.

  Note: These guidelines are not written in stone. Experiment with what works best for you. For example, the New York Knicks incorporate the following "three on; one off" variation:

  - Day 1: Ab power
  - Day 2: Ab fitness
  - Day 3: Ab strength
  - Day 4: Rest
  - Repeat

- Choose one to five exercises marked "ab power" in chapter 8.
- Oblique exercises work both sides of the body and therefore count as two exercises.
- Perform one to five sets of each exercise, 10 to 25 repetitions per set.
- Total repetitions during an ab power training session should not exceed 300.
- Since the purpose of this method of training is to develop power, don't focus on fatiguing the abdominals; rather, focus on performing each exercise explosively with maximum effort. Therefore, allow a minimum of one minute rest between sets.
- Be sure to include low back exercises—20 to 100 total repetitions. For the ab power level, choose one to five back exercises (or more if this is an area you wish to concentrate on). Do low back exercises marked "ab fitness," "ab strength," or "ab power," performing one to five sets of 5 to 20 repetitions.

Ab Power Sample Daily Routine

- **Maintain ab fitness level X two days per week.**
- **Maintain ab strength one to two days per week.**
- **Incorporate ab power one to two days per week.**

Ab Power Exercises	Sets*	Repetitions
1. Medicine Ball Snap Toss to a Wall (Left)	2	10
2. Medicine Ball Snap Toss to a Wall (Right)	2	10
3. Freestanding Knee-Ups	3	10
4. One-Seated Partner-Assisted Chest Pass Crunch	5	25

*Rest one minute minimum between each set.
Total repetitions per session: 195

Back Strength Exercises	Sets	Repetitions
1. Medicine Ball Back Crunch	3	10
2. Back Toss	3	10

TRAINING VARIATIONS

The regimens described in this manual are *not* etched in stone. Yet they have proven effective in developing abdominal toning, strength, and power. Even the best programs, however, can become monotonous or have their results stagnate after an extended period of time. If this is the case, vary the number of exercises, the repetitions, and the sets. For example, during an ab fitness routine, instead of 10 to 15 exercises, three sets of 15 repetitions, choose only 5 different exercises and perform several sets of 25 to 50 repetitions. Or choose 8 exercises and perform one set of 50 repetitions per exercise and so on. Each individual will respond differently to a particular program. Choose what works best for you.

GO AHEAD: IT'S WORTH IT!

One of the greatest concerns today is an overwhelming decline in physical fitness among people of all ages. With drastic budget cuts in education, the first to suffer are usually health curriculums, physical education, and intramural sports. Often shortsighted penny-pinching efforts eliminate entire athletic departments from school districts.

In a way, bureaucratic inefficiency is promoting a generation of unfit and health-ignorant youth.

It is a fact that considerable health benefits are associated with moderate levels of exercise for the general population. However, the weekend warrior, as well as the competitive athlete, requires more than just moderate levels of activity. *Stronger Abs and Back* bridges the gap between the general population and the elite athlete by providing abdominal routines that seriously challenge all individuals at any level.

Maybe you recognize that exercise is valuable but are so discouraged by the hard work and time commitment involved that you never get started on a program. But consider the specific benefits of exercise and overcome that inertia! Leading an active life will improve your stamina, your body composition, the overall functioning of your body, and, ultimately, your self-esteem. Still, training the center of power is but one component of the total training concept. Do not overlook the importance of cardiovascular efficiency, total body muscular strength and endurance, total body flexibility, and the elimination of unnecessary body fat when organizing your fitness training routine.

Initially, you may experience some physical discomfort, but this feeling will eventually be replaced by a positive transformation toward better health and, if you are so inclined, toward better athletic performance. Results, however, may not be immediate. Everyone responds to the training differently. You may improve rapidly or you may not see significant changes for several months. *But it will happen*, so don't give up. Certainly, developing optimal physical health is worth changing your lifestyle and investing the time and effort. Making the commitment and sticking with it will pay big dividends down the road.

About the Authors

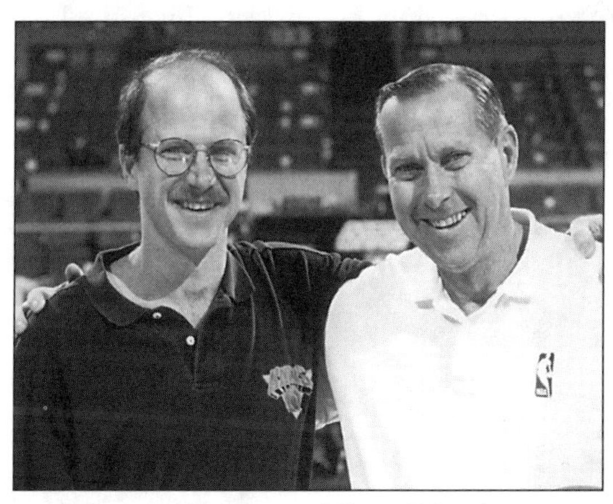

Greg Brittenham and Dean Brittenham

Dean Brittenham is the athletic director at the Shiley Athletic Elite Program at Scripps Clinic in La Jolla, California. He also is CEO of S.P.O.R.T. Elite, Ltd., an organization that promotes athletic performance, human health, and physical fitness through education, research, training, and service.

Dean Brittenham's background includes more than 40 years of teaching, training, and coaching athletes of all ability levels in many different sports. As a recognized expert in strength and conditioning, he is a popular speaker at camps, clinics, and symposia around the world. He has served as the strength and conditioning coach for both the Indiana Pacers and the New England Patriots, and he has trained a number of top-ranked tennis, volleyball, and cycling athletes.

Dean enjoys traveling, reading, and gardening. He lives in Escondido, California, with his wife, Beverly.

Greg Brittenham, Dean's son, is the strength and conditioning coach of the New York Knicks and has helped condition such NBA basketball pros as Patrick Ewing, Doc Rivers, and Derek Harper as well as players from the Orlando Magic and the Indiana Pacers. He also is the president of S.P.O.R.T. Elite, Ltd.

Greg has been a leader in athletic conditioning since 1978. He and his father were codirectors of the Center for Athletic Development at the National Institute for Fitness and Sport in Indianapolis. Greg holds a master's degree in kinesiology from Indiana University and is author of *Complete Conditioning for Basketball.*

An avid spokesperson for the importance of athletic conditioning, Greg has presented and demonstrated his training methods and programs to several prominent athletic groups, including the United States Tennis Association and the United States Olympic Committee. Greg lives in Stamford, Connecticut, with his wife, Luann, and their two children, Max and Rachel.